I0119188

The Great Escape
Love Duty and Defiance

Copyright © 2025 Philip A Webb

All rights reserved. No part of this publication may be reproduced or transmitted in any form or by any means, electronic or mechanical including photocopying, recording or any information storage or retrieval system, without prior permission in writing from the publishers.

The right of Philip A Webb to be identified as the author of this work has been asserted by him in accordance with the Copyright, Designs and Patents Act 1988

First published in the United Kingdom in 2025 by
The Cloister House Press

ISBN 978-1-78918131-01-7

Acknowledments

Adrian Umpleby, Burwell Christian home group, 2017/18
Joel and Sarah Dixon for their loving support, listenening to
my constant jabber, as they passed the gravy. We shall
treasure those days.
Richard and Joy Newman for their loyal friendship including
finding the perfect tenant for mum
as well as inviting mum and myself over for Sunday roast
dinners.
Munaza Ahmed who showed such trust and courage
throughout this "operation".
N.Tech. in Mansfield for carrying out the motorbility
modifications to my vehicle
Sue Cox, Angela's main carer at Midfield Lodge.
Lisa, Angela's personal carer at new home in Lowestoft.
Bill Calladine, my cousin who stronly suggested I write this
book.
Norfolk & Suffolk Social Services.
Christchurch Lowestoft for my continued belief and spiritual
grounding.

Contents

Chapter 1:

A Mother's Love:
Early Years In Cambridge

T he River Cam flows gently through Cambridge, carving stories into its banks just as surely as it carves channels through the ancient landscape. My story with my mother begins here, among the college punts and stone cottages that housed generations of scholars and townspeople alike.

Angela was born on March 2, 1933, in a small village called Landwade just north of Newmarket, six years before the Second World War would transform England forever. Her childhood unfolded in the quiet countryside, but she wasn't destined to remain there. At fourteen, she left the village schools behind and ventured to London with youthful determination, becoming a nanny for the family of Doctor Dean in Finchley.

London might have overwhelmed a lesser spirit, but Angela had a steadying influence nearby. Her uncle—my great uncle —lived close by in Ilford, providing a sanctuary when she wasn't working. She divided her time between the doctor's household and her uncle's home, building the foundation of independence that would later shape her mothering.

Life has its curious circles. While visiting Mrs. Vurnham—a kind woman who had looked after Angela when her own mother was hospitalized—she encountered the man who would become my father. They connected immediately, their chemistry undeniable, and on March 19, 1955, shortly after her twenty-second birthday, they married at Saint Giles Church in Cambridge.

The newlyweds settled into a cottage behind Northampton Street. It was there that I entered the world on September 1, 1956—their first and only child.

The cottage, though modest by today's standards, was our kingdom. We had no indoor bathroom, no plumbed bath— just a metal tub filled with water heated from a hob. My father worked long hours as an electrical engineer on the Comet jet, Britain's ambitious entry into commercial aviation. He also served in the Royal Electrical and Mechanical Engineers, often camping in Germany with the army, which meant his presence at home was precious but limited.

This absence created a special bond between my mother and me. We became co-conspirators, explorers, and sometimes adversaries in the small dramas of daily life. I was a spirited child with an irrepressible urge to escape our garden, climbing over a wall to play captain on the college punts moored nearby.

"He's down there!" neighbors would call, pointing toward the river as my mother emerged frantically from our cottage. The image remains vivid: Angela hurrying down to retrieve her wayward son, worry etched across her face.

My adventures weren't always innocent. Once, I hid close to the wall by the water, deliberately staying out of sight when she came looking. I could hear her gasping with fear as she scanned the river's surface. I chose that moment to pop my

2

head out, grinning impishly. She grabbed me, relief and anger competing in her voice: "Don't ever do that again! I thought you'd gone."

Such was our relationship—her constant care meeting my constant testing. It wasn't malice that drove my mischief but a child's delight in reaction, in being the center of her attention even when that attention came wrapped in worry.

When I was about four, our cottage life ended dramatically when the roof caved in. I was there when it happened, watching in terror as debris tumbled down the stairs. My mother's response was immediate and decisive: "That's it. We're out of here. We're not staying here any longer." Her protective instinct overrode any sentiment for our first home.

We moved to Kings Hedges Road, then on Cambridge's outskirts, surrounded by fields and farms—a stark contrast to our central location near the River Cam. The move marked a significant improvement in our living conditions. We now had proper bedrooms, a bathroom, and front and back gardens. My father enthusiastically landscaped the garden, growing vegetables and creating a family space. I remember the excitement of this new world opening before us.

In this expanded environment, my mother blossomed. She showed remarkable adaptability, joining neighborhood children for cricket on the foundations of houses under construction. Once, she fell into a concrete hole during a game, injuring her leg badly enough to confine her to bed for a time. This was typical Angela—fully engaged with life, unafraid to participate rather than merely supervise.

As I approached school age, she developed innovative ways to ensure I wouldn't be isolated as an only child. She discovered a family with horses and arranged for me to go riding each Saturday morning for half a crown per hour. Though this ended when my horse bolted with me—understandably terrified—it showed her commitment to broadening my experiences.

When horseback riding proved unsuitable, she redirected her efforts. Having noticed my friendship with Jeffrey, a boy with "a posh voice" she admired, she investigated and found he attended drama school. Soon, I was enrolled at the Mackenzie School of Drama for speech and elocution lessons. Angela was determined I would have advantages she hadn't, including refined speech and cultural exposure.

Not all these efforts met with my enthusiasm. I flatly refused to enter ballet school, pressing my feet against the door when she tried to lead me inside, mortified by the room full of girls visible through the window. Her aspirations and my resistance created a delicate dance of wills throughout my childhood.

Angela found ways to contribute to the household income as our circumstances improved. She established a hairdressing salon in our home, building a clientele through word of mouth as the neighborhood around us grew from fields to a thriving community. Clients—many of them mothers of my school friends—would arrive to have their hair "done" while I would slip past, heading to the kitchen with a casual "I'm starving."

Angela possessed an exceptional eye for beauty and design. Everything she chose for our home reflected a thoughtful selection, from furniture to decorative objects. This aesthetic sensibility extended to her personal appearance. Though never heavily made-up, she was strikingly beautiful when she applied makeup for special occasions. Her taste in clothing was impeccable—she knew instinctively what suited her and our home.

An unexpected influence came through a university graduate and artist named Victor Ramsthoff, who used a shed beside our former property as his studio. It became his workspace, and he and Angela formed a friendship that would last throughout their lives.

Victor came from "somewhere east of Suez"—a phrase that captured his exotic difference in our provincial setting. He provided companionship for Angela during my father's frequent absences, bringing artistic perspectives into our home.

Interestingly, I sometimes called my mother "Angela" rather than "Mum." This habit developed after visiting my mother's brother in Newmarket, where I noticed my cousins called their mother by her first name. The practice stuck, and throughout my life, I alternated between the formal "Angela" and the intimate "Mum," depending on my mood and the situation.

My relationship with "Mum" wasn't only defined by my mischief or her care. One poignant memory involves a Saturday morning when choosing to hunt for conkers on Victoria Avenue instead of attending my drama lesson; I lost the envelope containing the entire term's fees for Drama School.

Angela, our neighbor Jim Rolph, and I searched for hours that afternoon, but the money had vanished. I harbored suspicions about my friend Jeffrey but couldn't prove anything. The incident taught me about responsibility and consequences in a way no lecture could have.

Through these early years in Cambridge, Angela shaped my world not just through practical care but also through her values, aesthetic sense, social connections, and ambitions for me. As an only child, I was the focus of her considerable energy and attention. Though I often tested her patience, the foundation she laid during those formative years built a connection that would sustain us through the much more difficult challenges that lay ahead.

Looking back, I see now that the cottage behind Northampton Street and the house on Kings Hedges Road weren't just places we lived—they were spaces where Angela created a world for us, brick by brick and moment by moment, through the steady application of a mother's love.

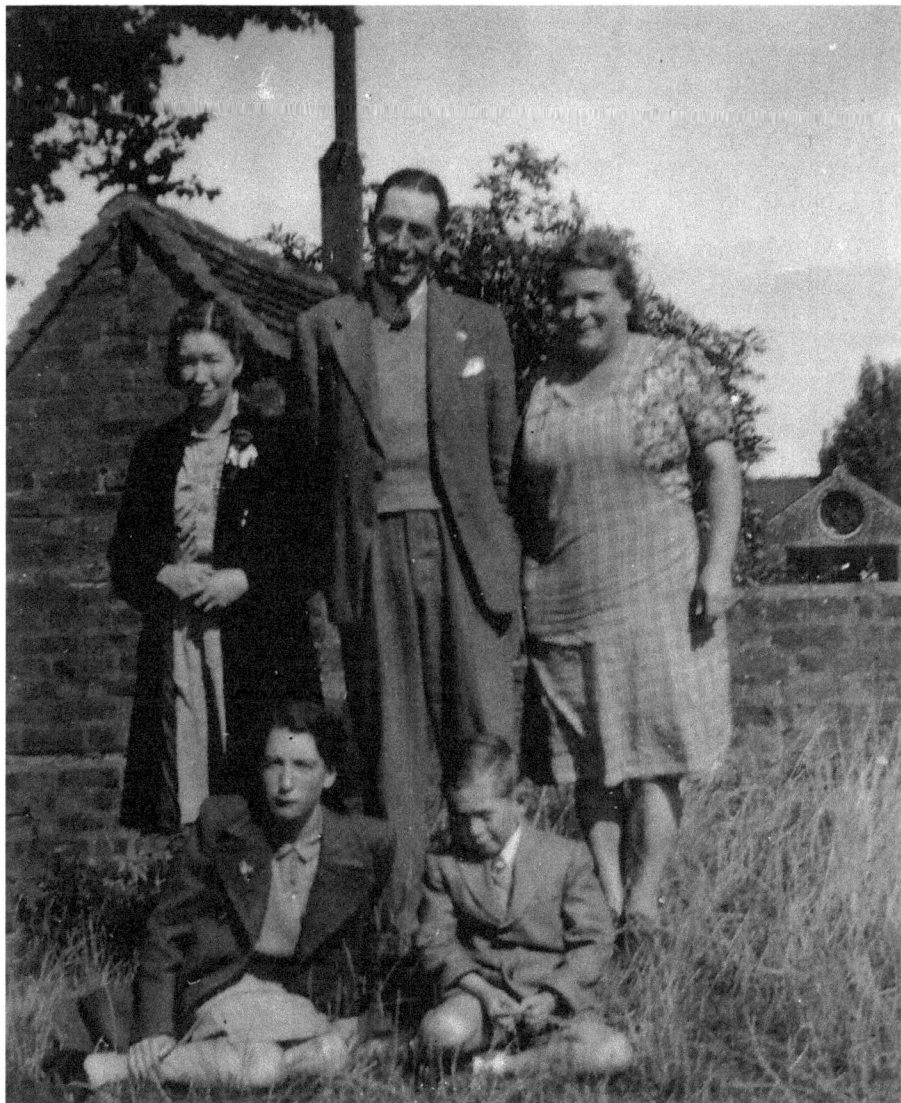

*Angela beside her young brother John. Florence far left and Fred Archer
above. Landwade, Newmarket.*

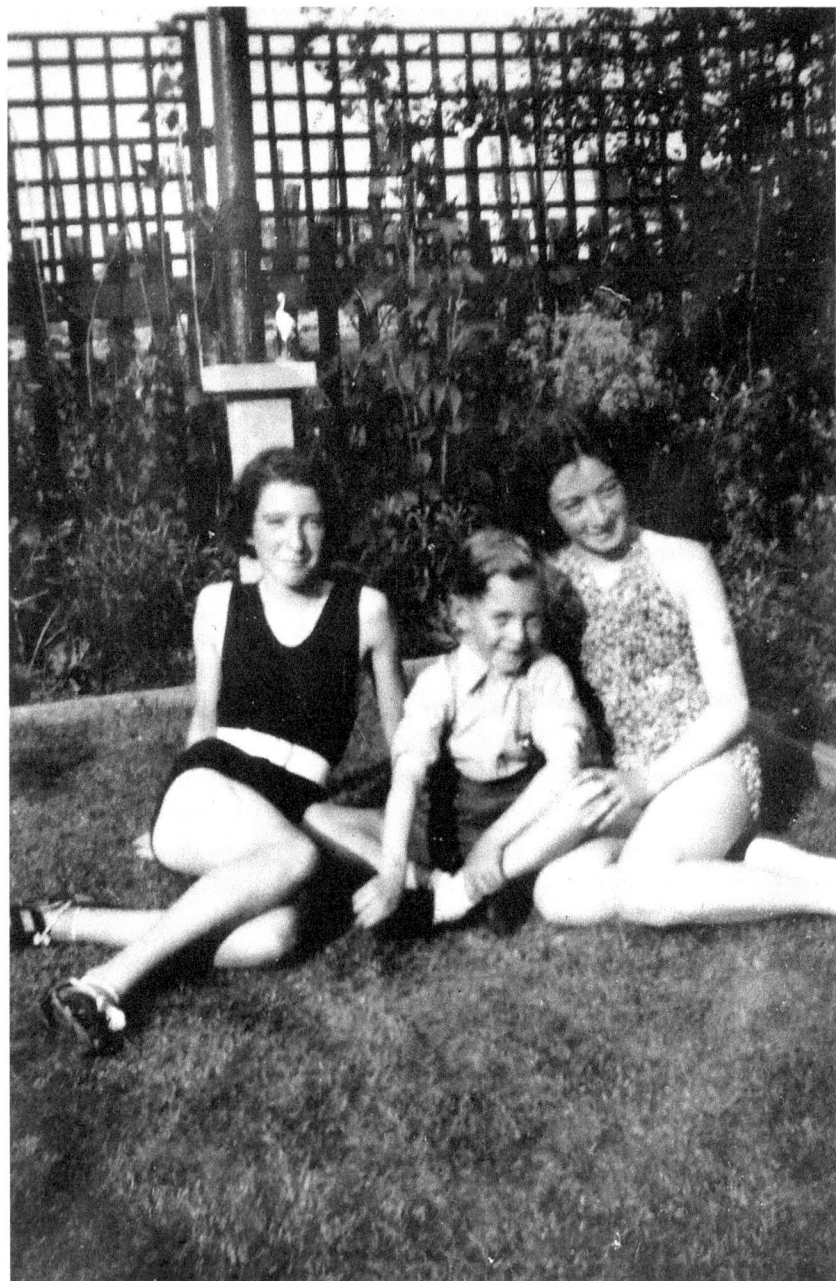

Angela together with brother John and sister Thelma in her Uncle's rear garden, Newbury Park, Ilford, Essex. 1945 circa.

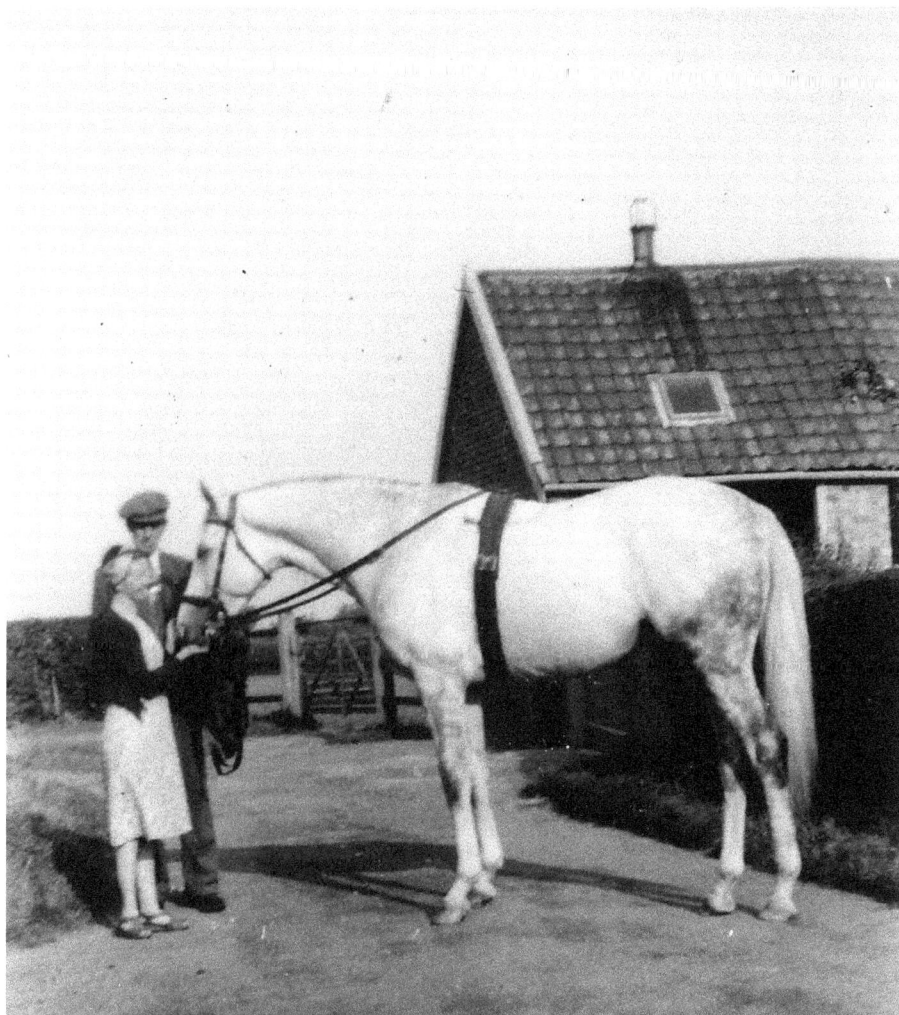

Fred Archer (no relation to the jockey), horseman to Epsom Derby winner Airborne. Photo 1946 with proud wife Florence.

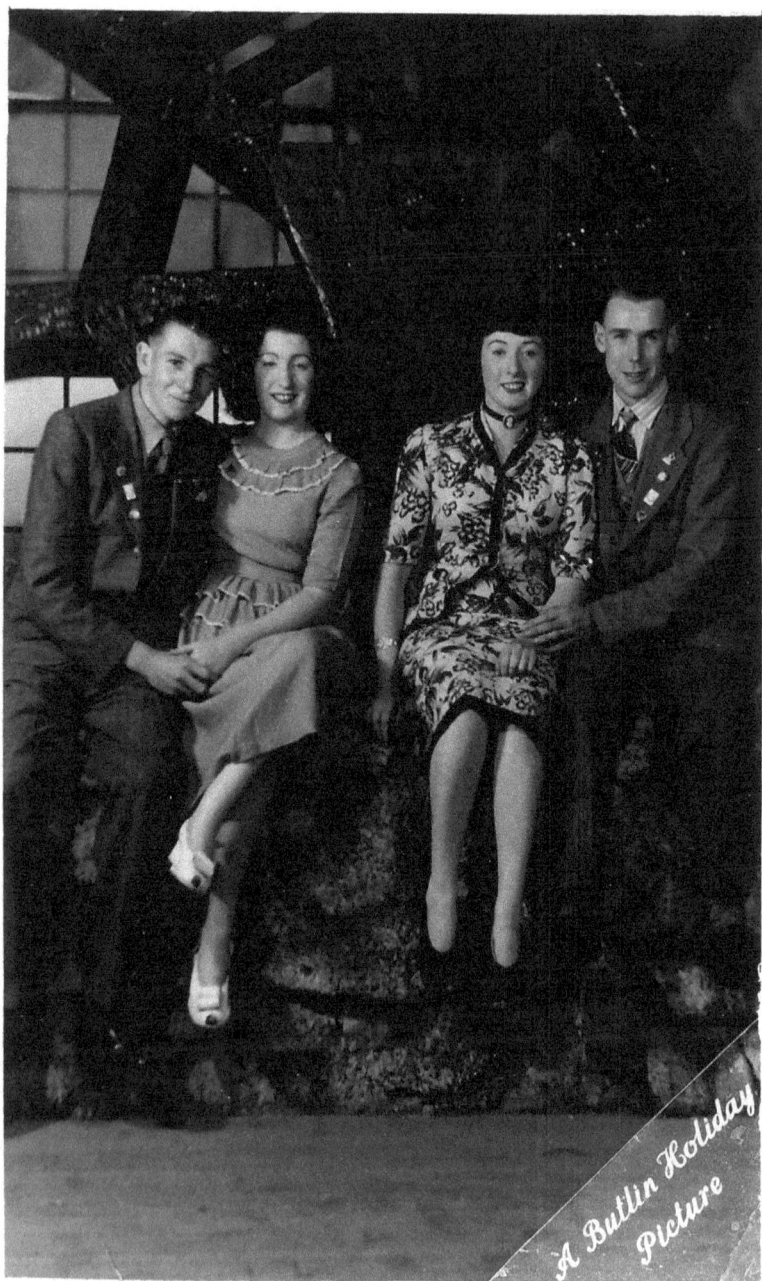

The two sisters seen here out having fun with American servicemen at Butlins Holiday Park. Photo circa 1949.

10

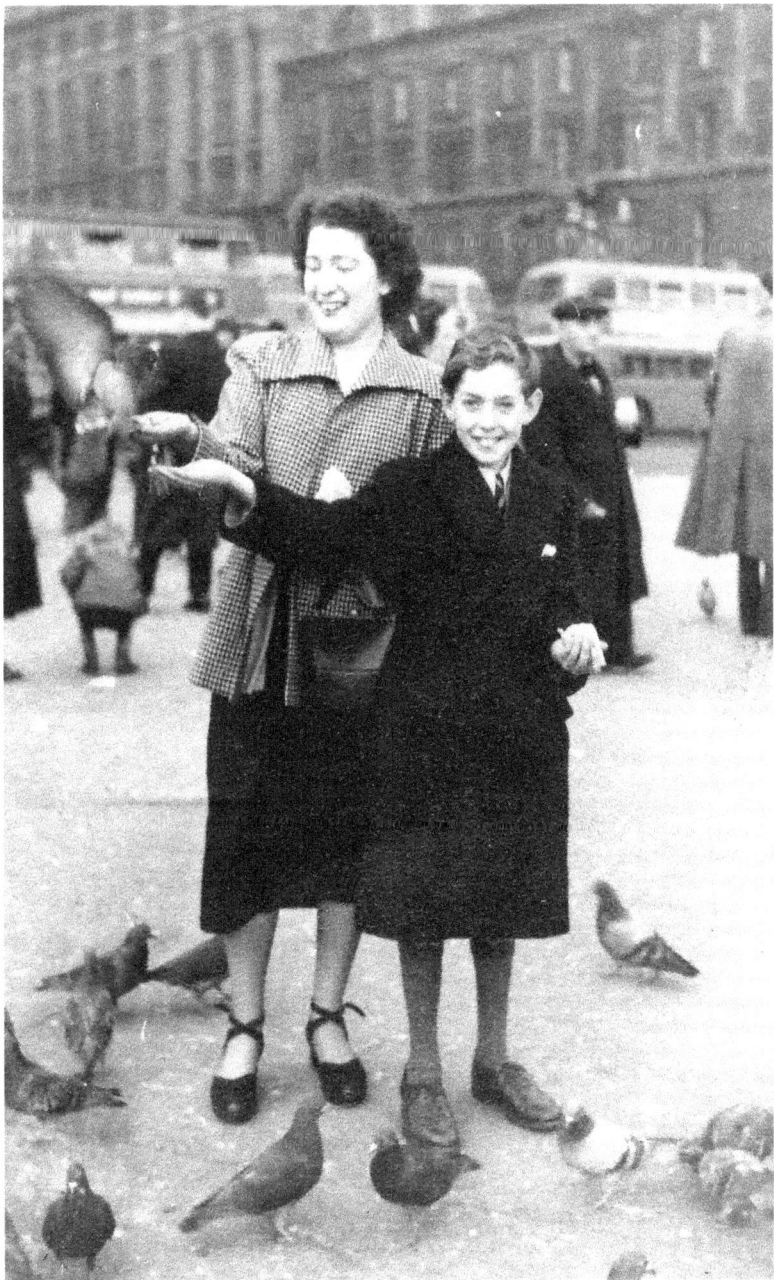

Angela with her brother John out in London. Now in Full employment with Doctor Deans family in Finchley. 1950.

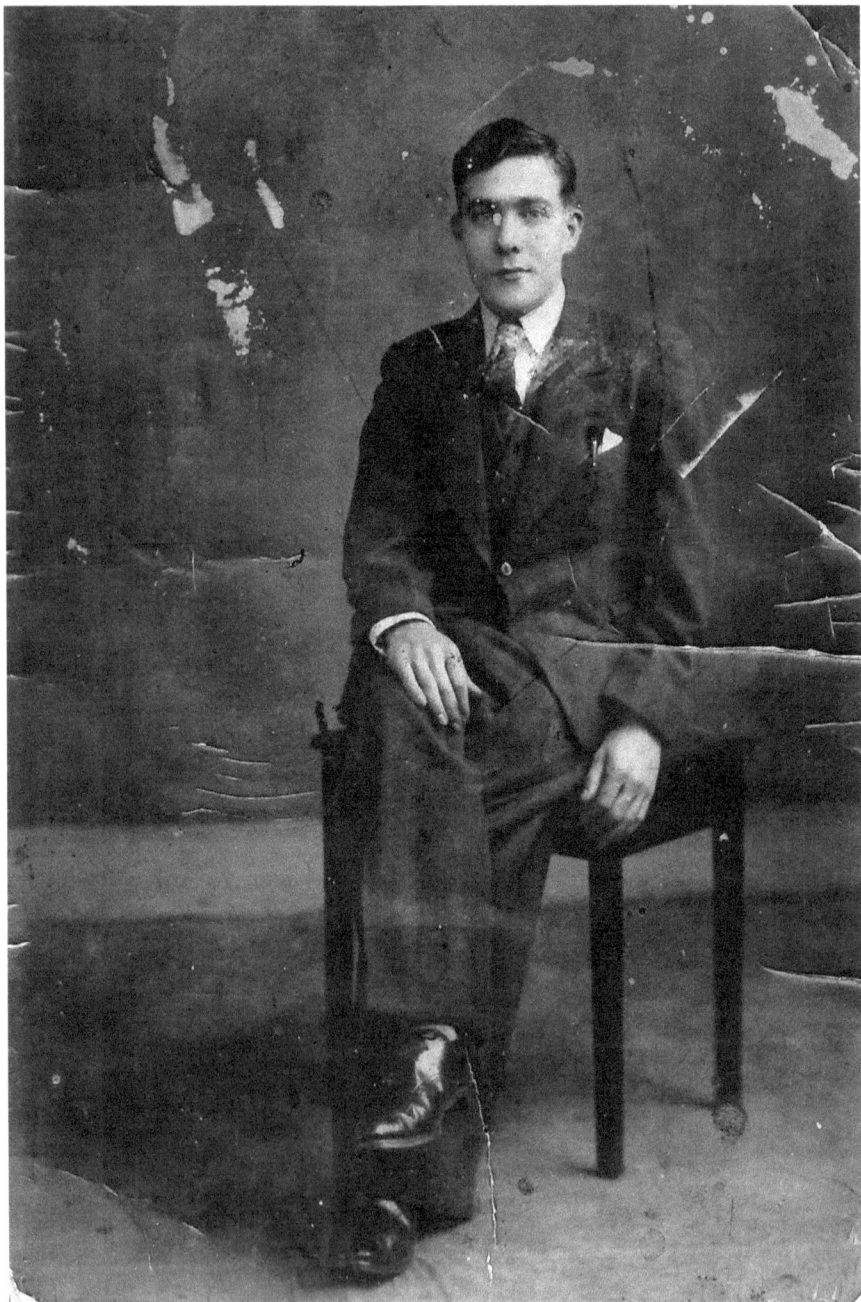

Stanley (Sam) Webb. Angela's Husband to be.

12

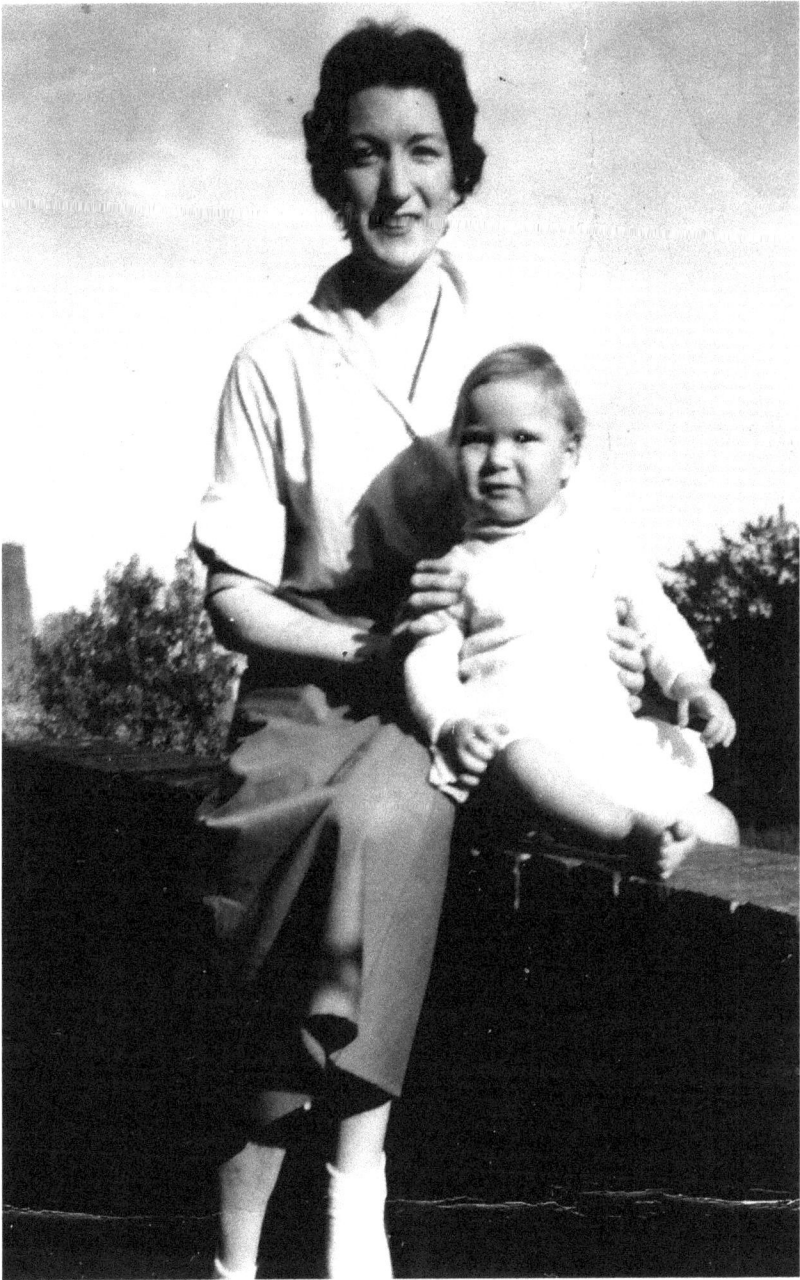

With Philip after his Christening (baptism) in St. Gile's Church, Cambridge.
CB3 0AQ. Photo 1956.

13

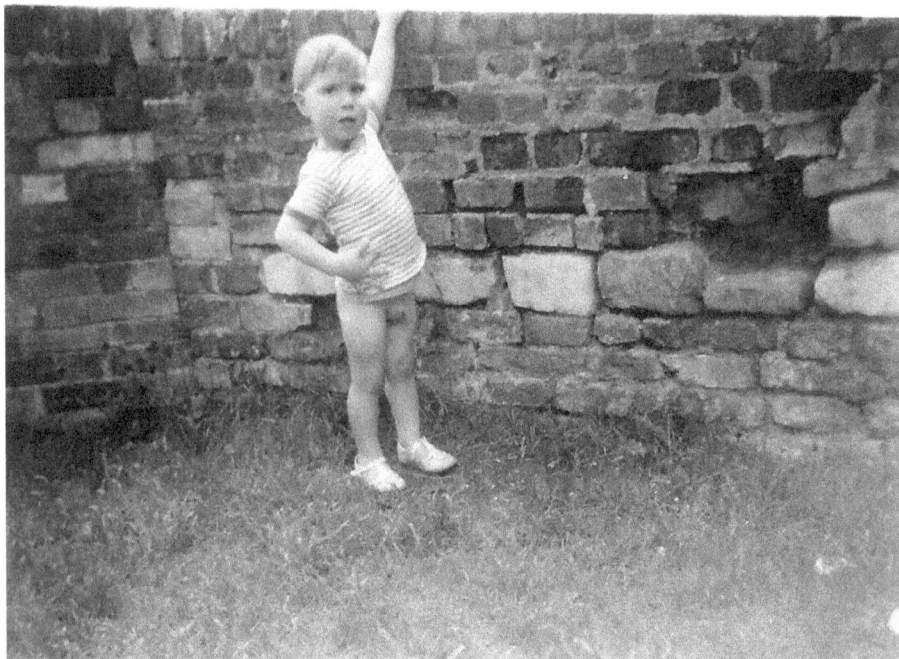

The garden wall at 2 Gentle's Yard which was to keep Philip home safe while Angela attended to all the housework. 1957.

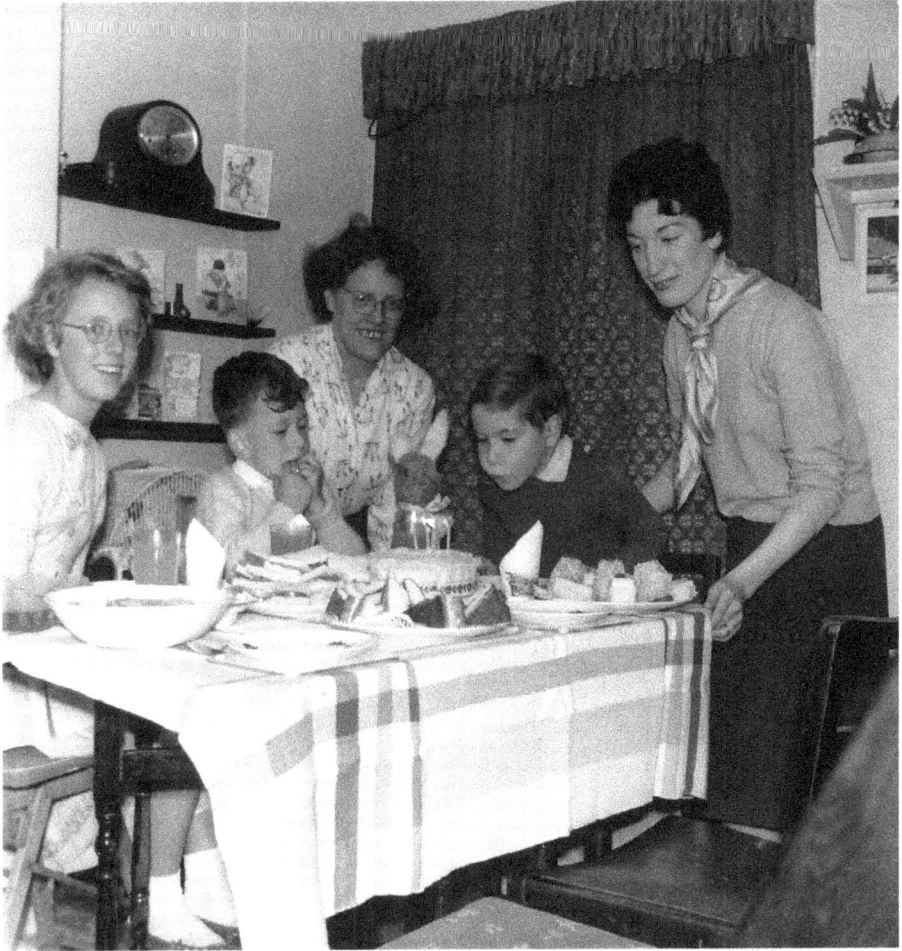

Phil's 4th Birthday at the cottage in Gentle's Yard. At table are Gill, Billy as their mother Betty and Angela look on.

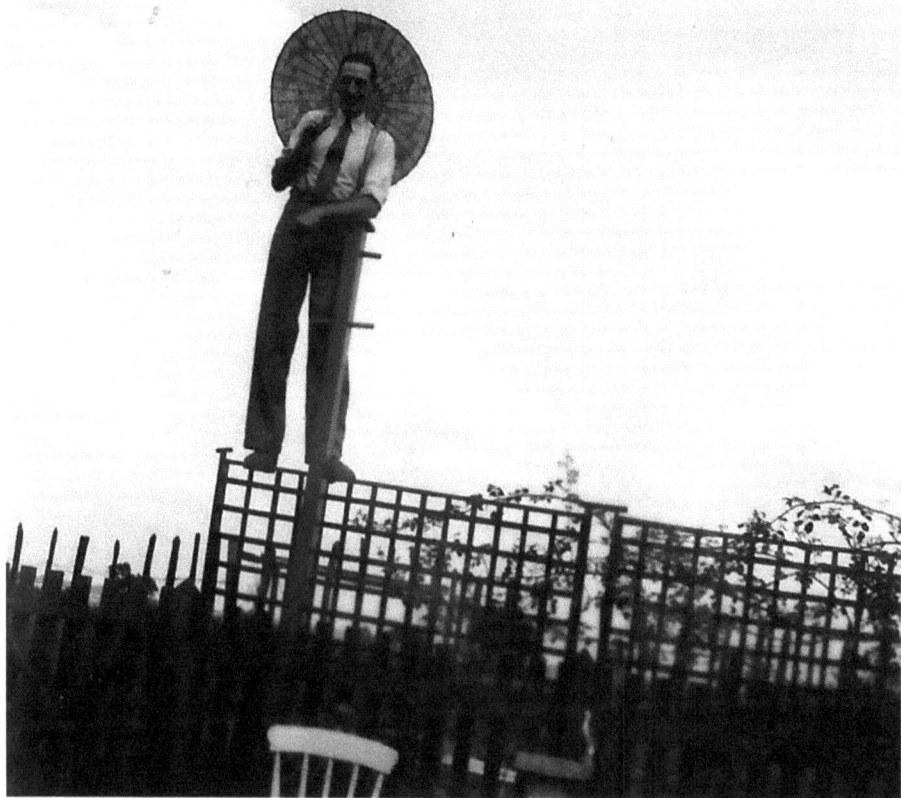

Mum's dad, Fred, larking about at Unle Ern's. Always a great character with heaps of spontaneous stimuli to entertain.

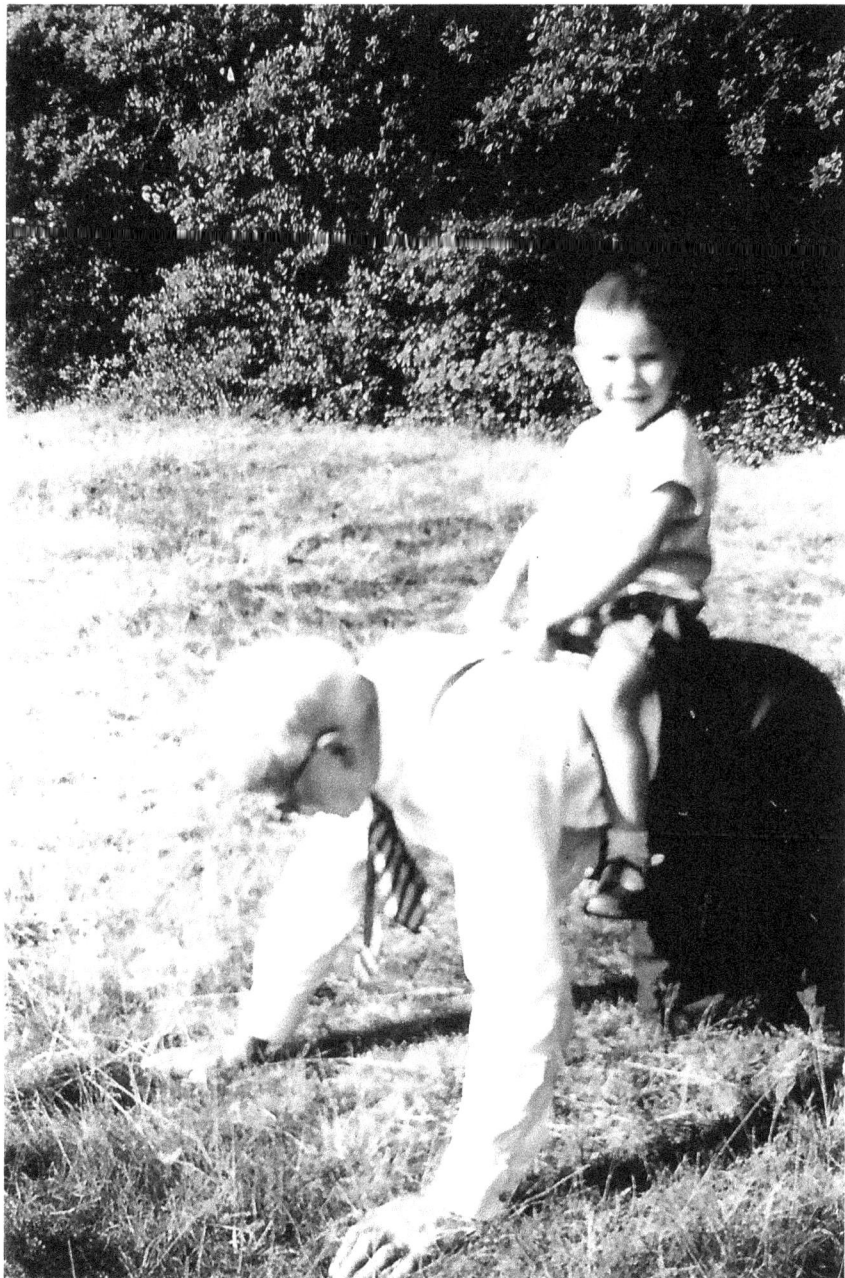

Riding along on Uncle's back. The early days of exuberance, in parks, his allotment, museums, theaterland...endless joy.

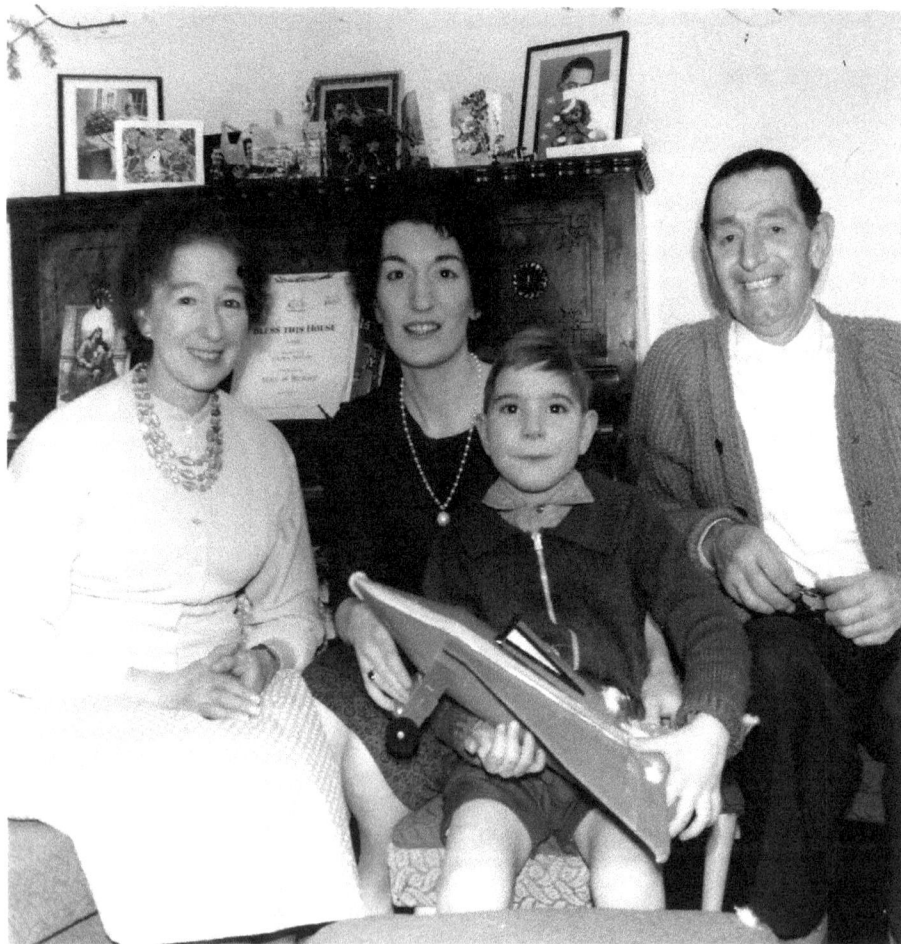

Angela with her Mum Florry, her Dad and Philip with his birthday present from his grandparents. Circa 1960.

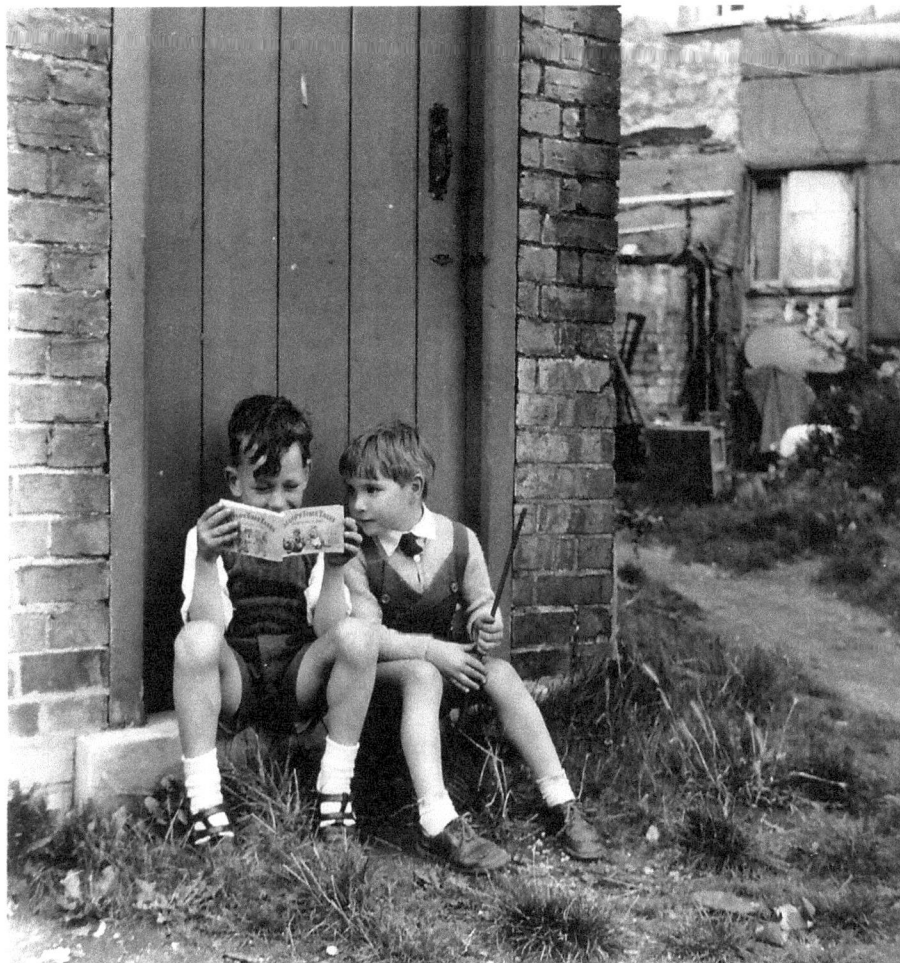

Gentle's Yard, Cambridge: the big step to the outside privy makes a good seat for Billy and me. circa 1960.

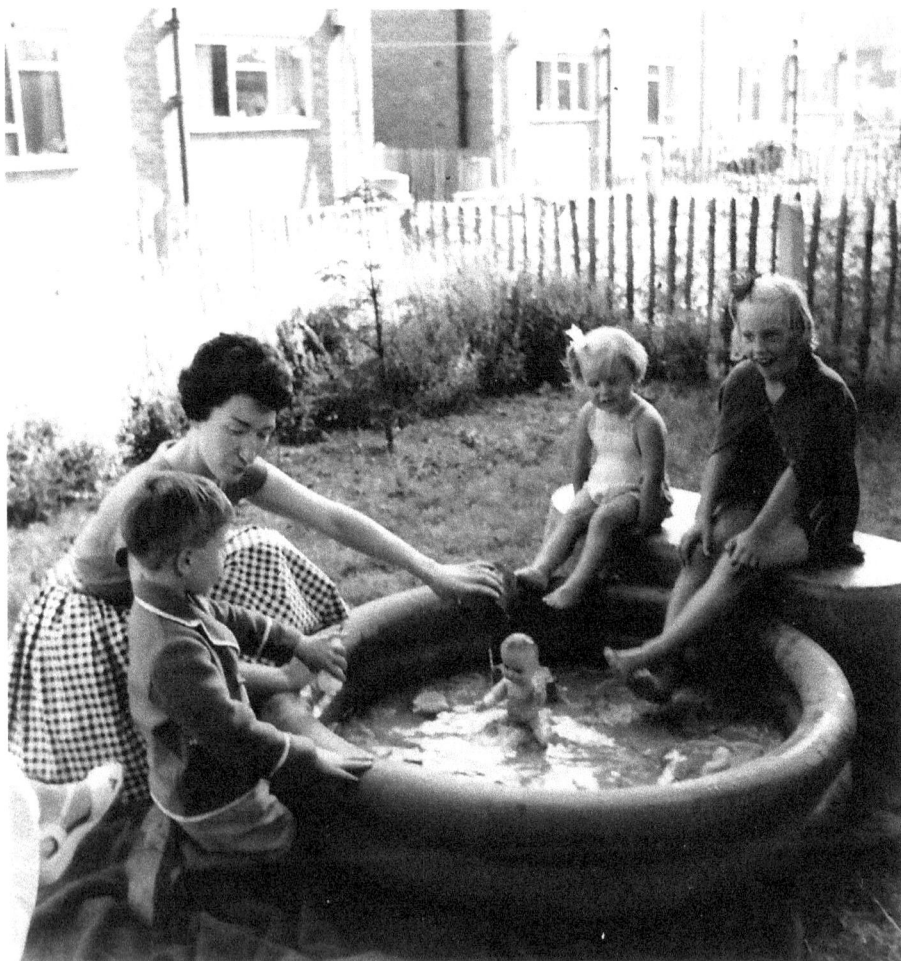

*Angela encourages Phil to play, except Phil is far from keen on paddling pools,
girl talk and their dolls. Stetchworth.*

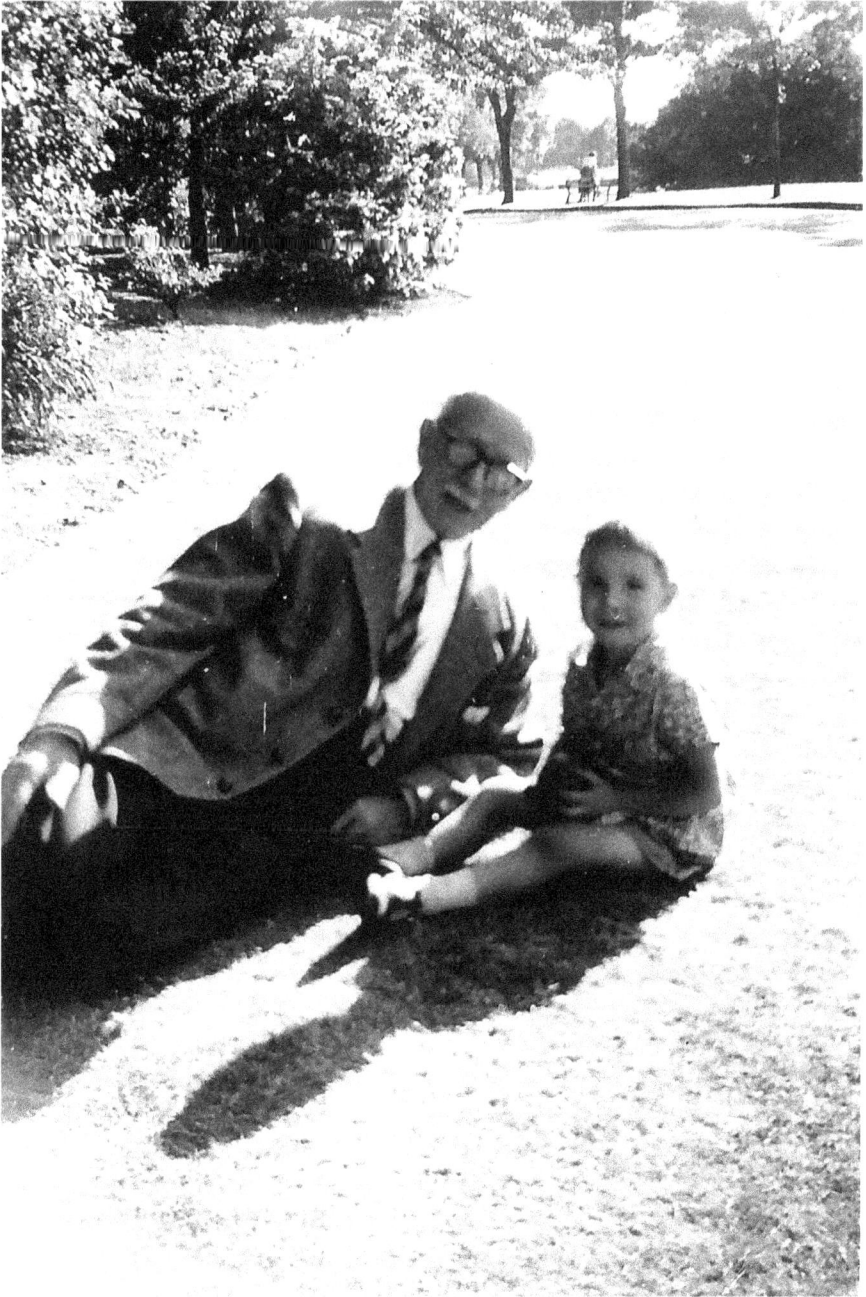

Philip with Gt. Uncle Ernest in Valentines Park. Photo by Angela 1959.

21

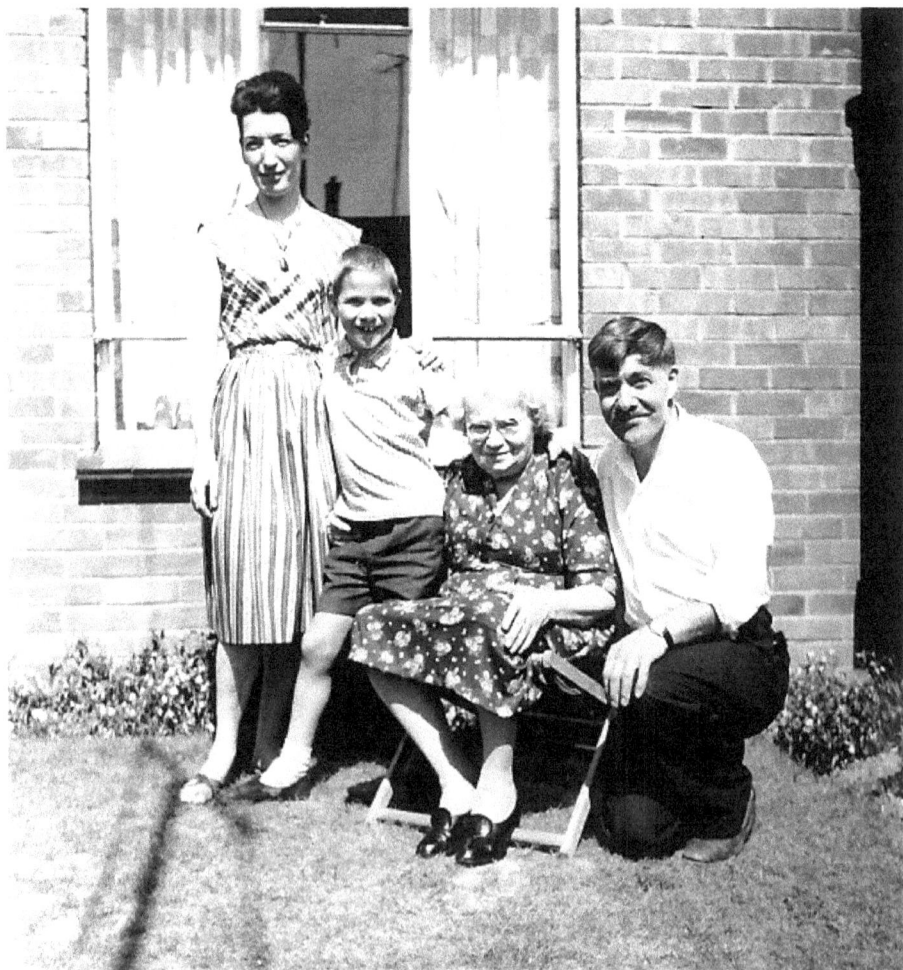

Grandma Webb comes to visit us at our new house, 91 King's Hdg's. 1963.

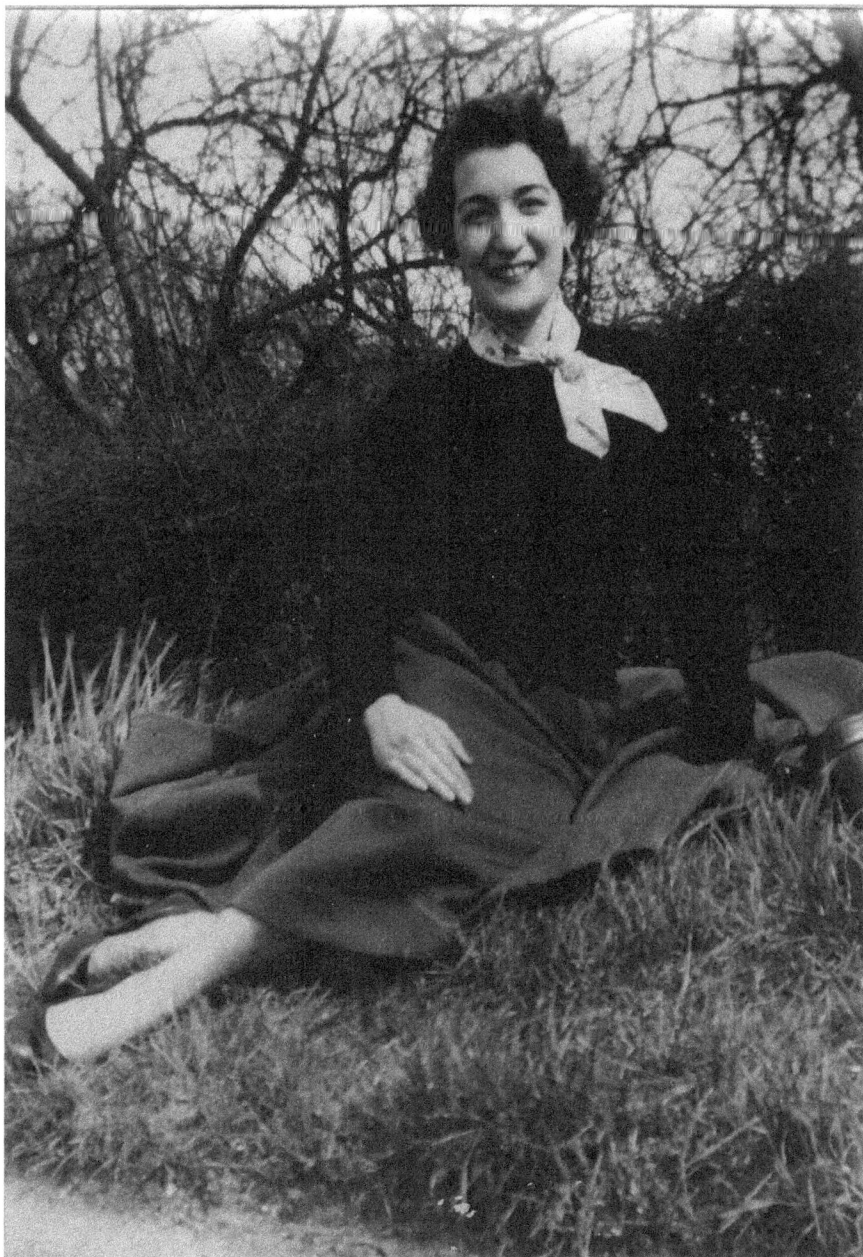

Before Philip came into the world, there were many long country walks around Stetchworth with Sam.

23

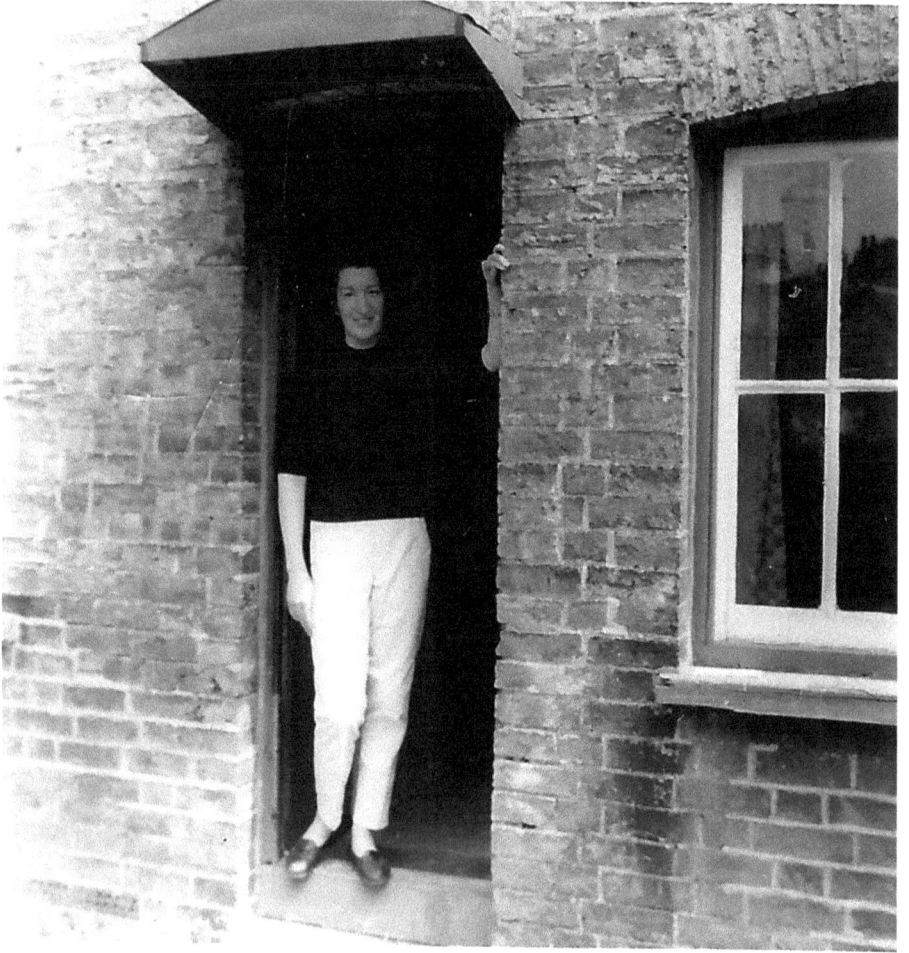

Our first house, the cottage behind Northampton Street, No. 2 Gentle's Yard. situated behind the Pickeral public house.

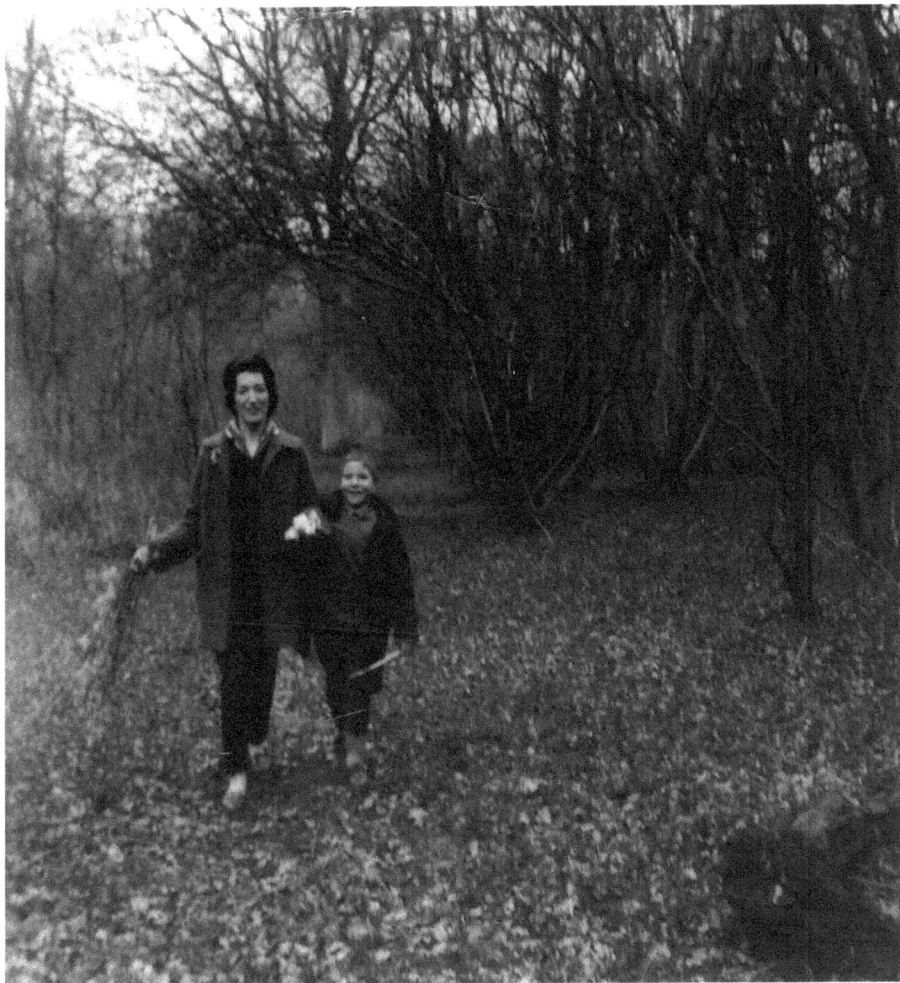

walking together through Hainault Forest during autumn. Photo by Uncle Ernie. 1964

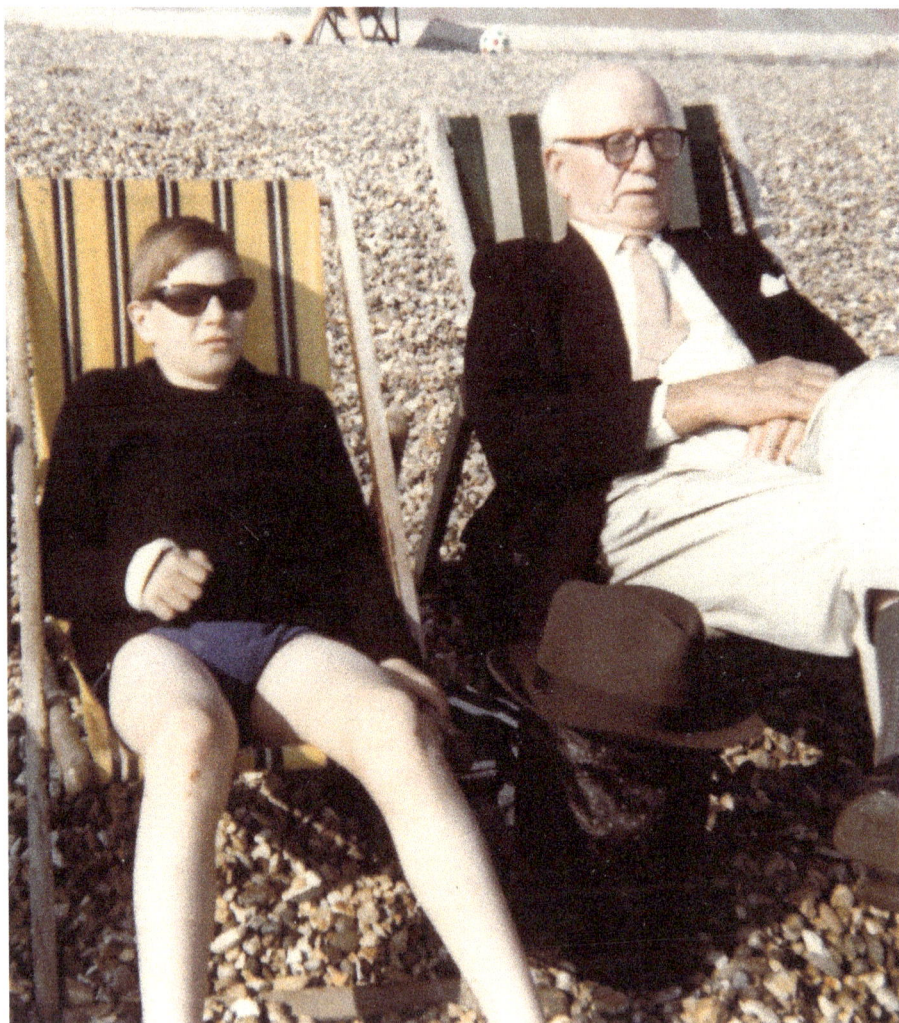

Uncle Ernie and Phil still with his arm in plaster. Taken by Angela on holiday at Walton on the Naze, 1965

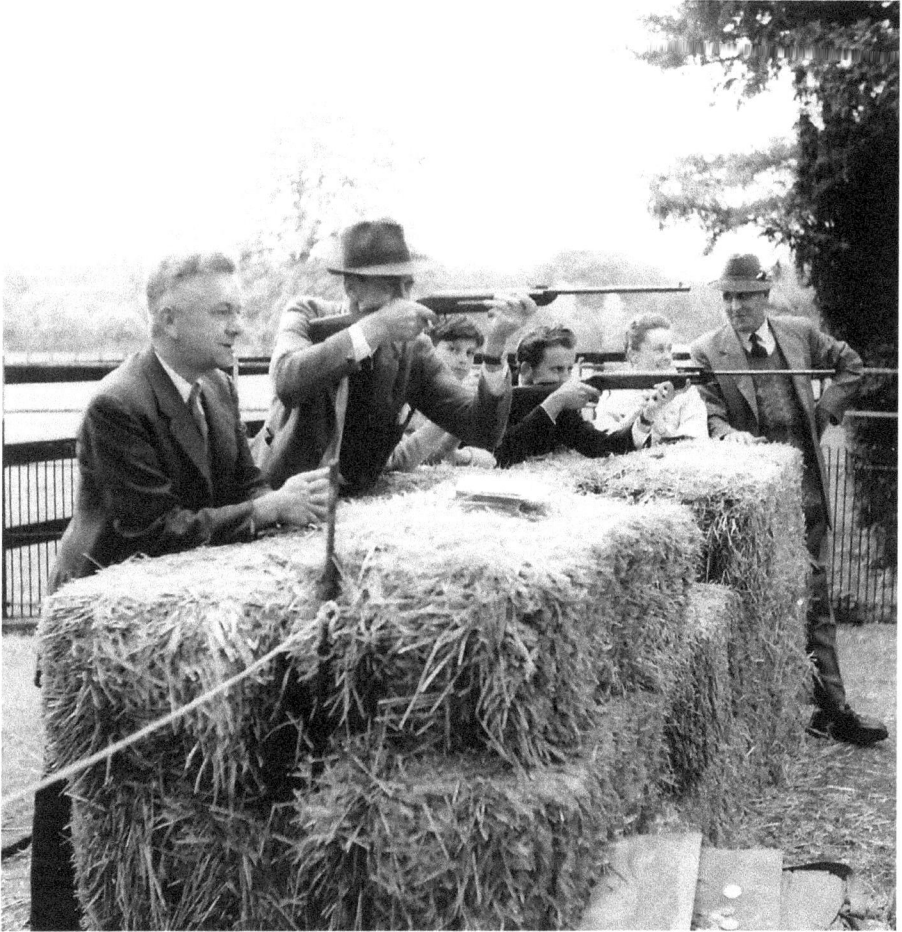

Grandad Fred was also a crack shot. He would take me out shooting during the summer holidays on the land.

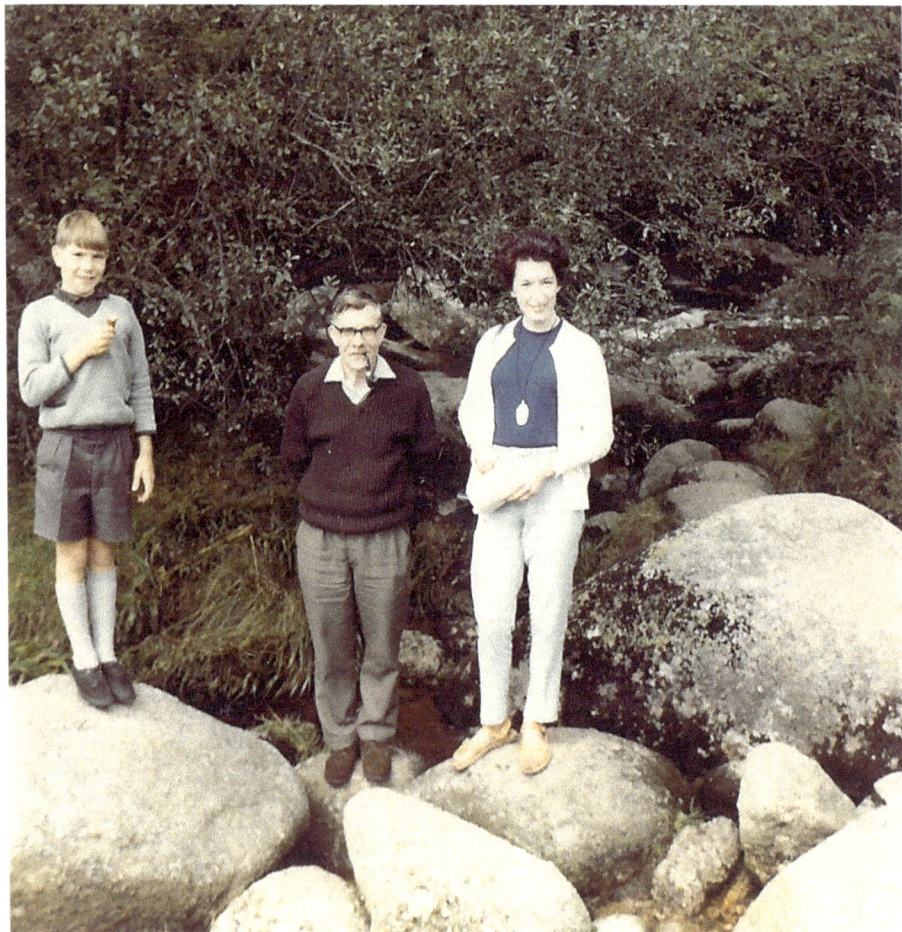

One of many holidays spent in Devon. Angela now paid for a man to come on holiday with us, known as Jim the driver. 1964

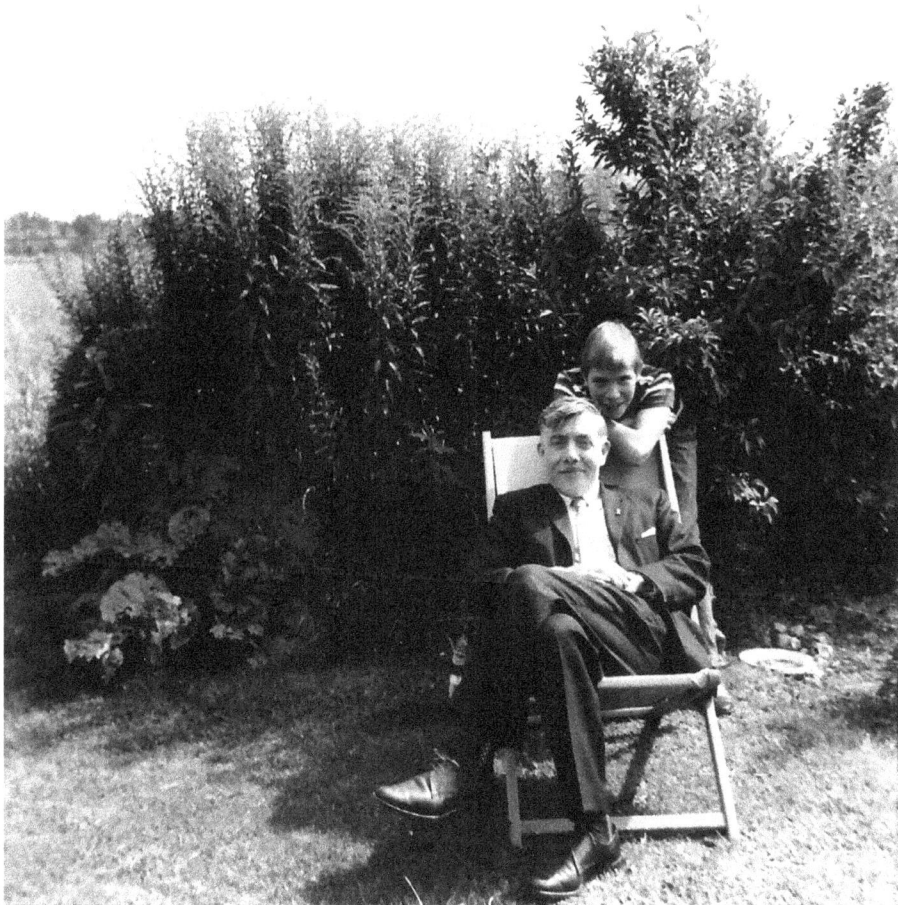

Sam and Phil enjoying the sun in the garden of Grandma and Grandad's in Stetchworth, Suffolk. 1965.

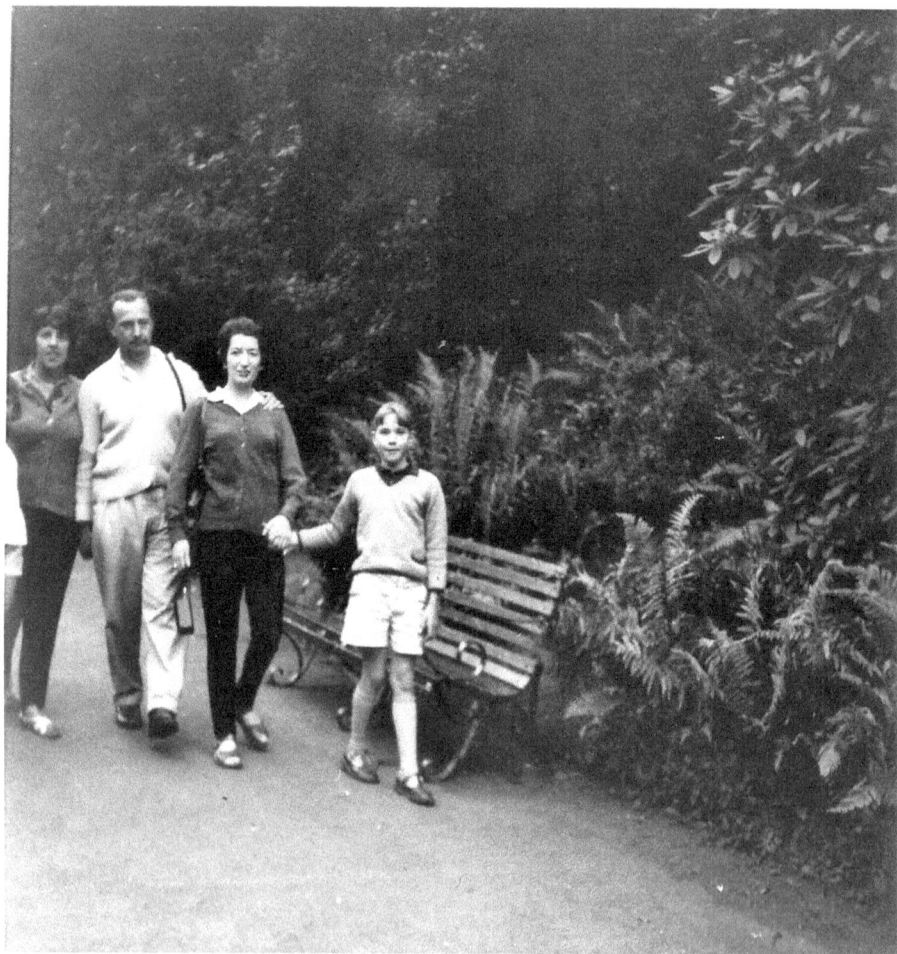

This time a holiday in Devon with the Rudd family, by now Phil was listening to pop music, particulay The Rolling Stones

Chapter 2:

Growing Up Together:
A Mother's Guidance

The summer of 1966 stretched before me like an endless promise. Golden afternoon light spilled across football pitches where I, at nine years old, captained the Grove County Junior School team to victory after victory. Something magical crystallized that year—a perfect alignment of childhood ambition and achievement that remains forever preserved in my memory.

I can still feel the weight of responsibility as I led our team to the triple cup, winning every match against competing schools. More than just a team captain, I was also our top goal scorer. Such prominence on the pitch translated to social status in the playground—I had girlfriends, admirers, and a sense of belonging that seemed to validate my entire existence.

Beyond our school triumphs, the nation itself was caught in football fever. When England won the World Cup that summer, my personal victories seemed cosmically connected to something larger. This was my golden year—the standard against which I would measure the seasons of my life to come.

Grove County Junior was a brand-new mixed school, a refreshing environment where I thrived after leaving the oppressive Victorian building of my first educational experience. My mother had been concerned when I started school, especially as she'd been ill when my great uncle took me for my first day. I landed in the wrong class and wandered the halls confused, already in trouble on day one. But at Grove County, everything changed. The teachers liked me; I liked them. The clean modernity of the building offered fresh possibilities.

Our family circumstances had improved, too. My mother's hairdressing clientele had increased and my father found a new job with Simplex, an agricultural manufacture, out at Sawston. Life had a comfortable rhythm.

Summer holidays meant Folkestone, where someone in our wider family owned a holiday house we rented for two weeks each year. These escapes from Cambridge's routine became the canvas for a mother's creative parenting. Sensing my growing curiosity about the wider world, she nurtured my budding independence.

During the 1966 holiday—that magical summer—I relentlessly badgered my parents about taking the ferry to France. My father resisted, but I had developed persuasive skills beyond my years.

"We haven't got passports," my parents protested.

"Yes, but you can get day passports," I countered, having researched this myself.

For every obstacle they raised, I'd discovered a solution. Eventually, they relented, and we crossed the Channel—my first international adventure, engineered through sheer determination and my mother's willingness to embrace my dreams.

Angela later conspired with me to send a postcard to my school, which arrived perfectly timed with my return after our two-week absence. My teacher read it aloud to the class while I covered my face in mortification—a moment of public attention engineered by Angela's mischievous support.

These holidays offered more than recreation. At Folkestone, I encountered a sign writer working in his shop, meticulously crafting letters with fluid precision. Something clicked as I watched him work—here was my future, revealed in careful brushstrokes and perfect spacing. From age nine onward, I nurtured this career ambition for five years. Mother encouraged it, saying, "Let's stick to that." She recognized the importance of a child finding their direction.

Years later, the devastation was profound when a careers advisor dismissed my dream, declaring sign writing "a dead trade." In that moment of casual discouragement, something fundamental shifted in my educational trajectory. My previously promising school performance began to deteriorate. Without realizing it, this advisor had extinguished a guiding light, leaving me adrift just as I entered the turbulent waters of adolescence.

The transition from Grove County Junior to senior school marked another painful rupture. After the bright, mixed environment I'd loved, I found myself confined to an all-boys institution separated from the girls' school by a towering wall —"like East Germany and West Germany," with supervised separation that felt archaic and punitive. Gone was the camaraderie of the football pitch and the easy social navigation of mixed classes. This new environment demanded a different kind of survival.

A clerical error compounded my difficulties. Born on September 1st, I should have been the oldest in my class, but instead was placed a year ahead, making me the youngest. This administrative oversight would follow me throughout my education, leaving me perpetually out of sync with my peer group.

My academic performance, once promising, deteriorated into rebellion. I tested boundaries, challenged teachers, and joined a gang where some members eventually landed in prison. We weren't feral—we were intelligent boys making poor choices. By fourteen, I'd had enough. While others in my class prepared for O-levels, I announced my intention to leave school.

My father, military background evident in his rigid posture, delivered an ultimatum: "If you don't come back home within a week with a job, you're not living here anymore."

I walked into a construction company office the next day. "I want to be an electrician," I told them.

"We don't have that, but we can offer you a painting and decorating apprenticeship," they replied.

Just like that, I'd secured a four-year apprenticeship that might eventually lead to becoming a tradesman. My father couldn't argue with employment, though it wasn't the art college I'd secretly hoped for.

At fifteen, too young to properly begin my apprenticeship, I spent six months merely observing journeymen, sweeping up after them, and absorbing the basics of the trade. The structure felt both confining and aimless after the focus of my sign-writing ambition.

By seventeen, restlessness had taken hold. I hitchhiked from Cambridge to Wales, catching the ferry from Holyhead to Ireland, testing my independence and measuring the world beyond our neighborhood. A year later, I took a more ambitious journey, boarding the Istanbul Express for a three-day adventure across Eastern Europe to the gateway between continents. The experiences expanded my horizons but did nothing to settle my internal turbulence.

Upon returning to England, I refused to go back to work, a behavior my mother recognized as concerning. She took decisive action, bringing me to a psychiatric hospital where I would spend six months—a period that felt like a necessary pause, a sabbatical from the building pressures of early adulthood.

I needed to get away and sort everything out and try and make sense of what was going on with my life, I realize now, looking back.

It was a time to reset, supported by my mother's unflinching practicality in the face of mental health challenges.

After my hospital stay, Angela's networking abilities revealed themselves again. She spoke with friends, the Rolfes, who ran a fuel company delivering oil to homes. Through this connection, I found work—another stepping stone arranged through her quiet intervention.

My entrepreneurial spirit eventually emerged. I bought a motorcycle, passed my test, and started working as a dispatch rider for a courier company. Within a few years, I established my own courier business, which I later sold to focus on new ventures. By twenty-six, I had purchased a one-bedroom flat in Cambridge, a tangible symbol of independence that surprised even my mother.

Her pride when she saw how I had decorated it confirmed what I'd always sensed—beneath her worries lay a fundamental belief in my potential.

The business flourished despite her concerns about my safety. Her prayers followed me along the highways and byways —justified anxiety, as I did suffer one serious accident. Yet she never demanded I stop, understanding that I needed to find my own path, even with its risks.

By my late twenties, a pattern had emerged in our relationship. Angela worried I pushed boundaries, yet we remained tethered by mutual respect. Even during my most rebellious phases, I recognized the solid foundation she had built—a base from which I could launch myself into adventures, knowing there was always a place to return.

Her guidance came not through lectures but through consistent presence, practical support, and an unwavering faith that, eventually, I would find my way. She balanced protection with permission, creating space for me to make mistakes while ensuring those mistakes wouldn't be catastrophic.

The boy who once jumped onto college punts against her wishes had grown into a young man who crossed continents on his own. Through it all, Angela adjusted her mothering to my changing needs—never abandoning her core principles but adapting how she expressed them as I matured. It was a dance of increasing distance and enduring connection, choreographed with imperfect steps but genuine love.

Together, we were growing up—mother and son, each learning from the other how to navigate the unpredictable currents of an ordinary, extraordinary life.

The dream team in a dream year 1966 Triple Cup winners

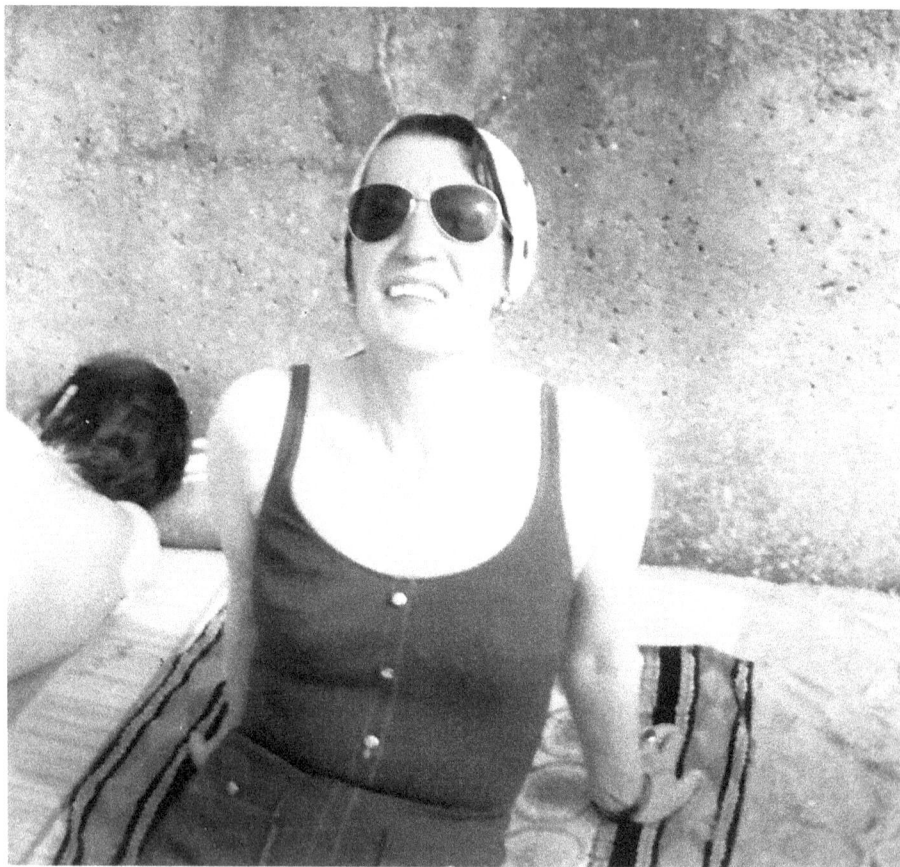

A much treasured get-a-way, taking Phil with them after his dicharge from hospital.

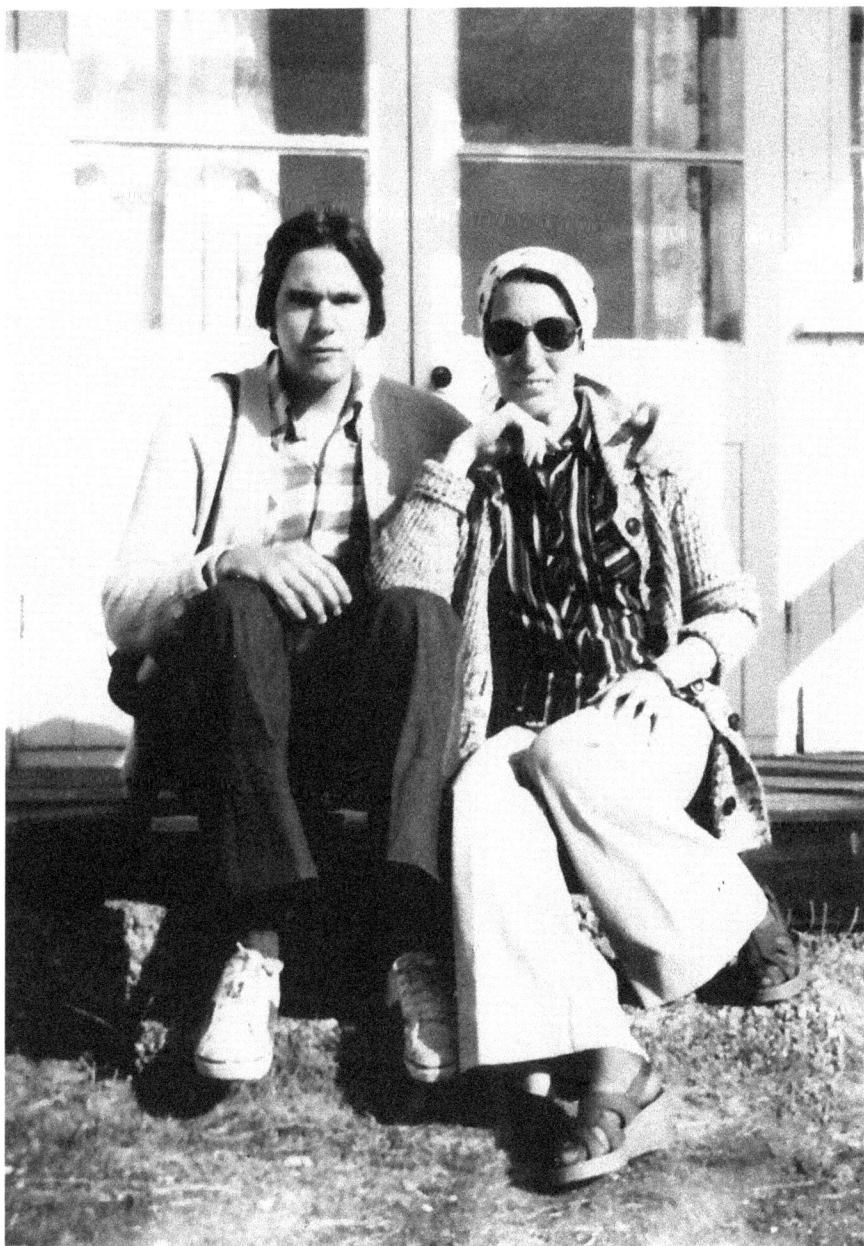

East coast in a caravan owned by the Rolphs. Angela supporting Phil as he tries to recover. Photo circa 1977.

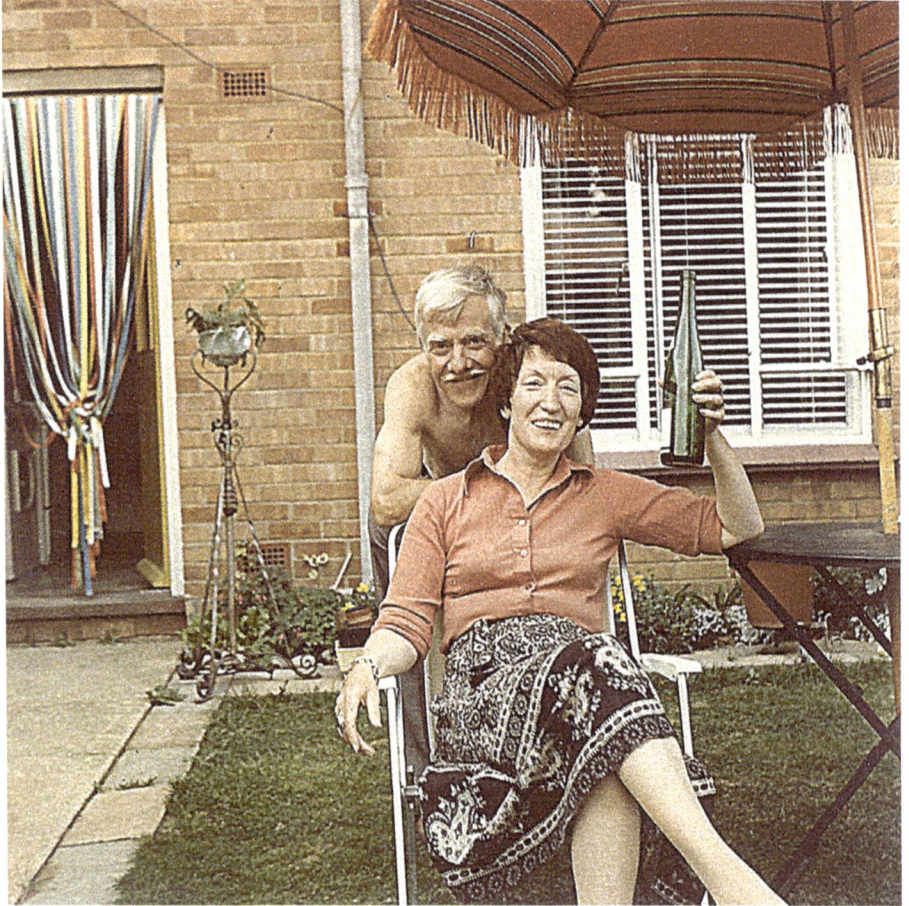

Angela and Sam succseffully buy the freehold of the house they'd been renting for 20 years. Now its rent free time. 1980

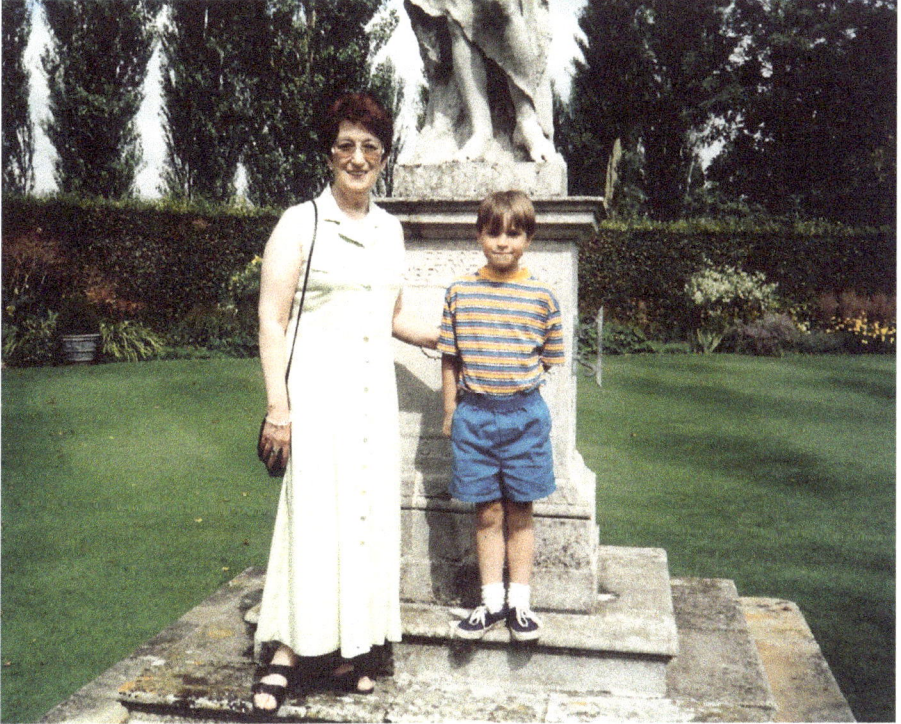

Angela with one of many meetings with Austin her beloved grandson. He was adopted at Phil's request as Phil became ill.

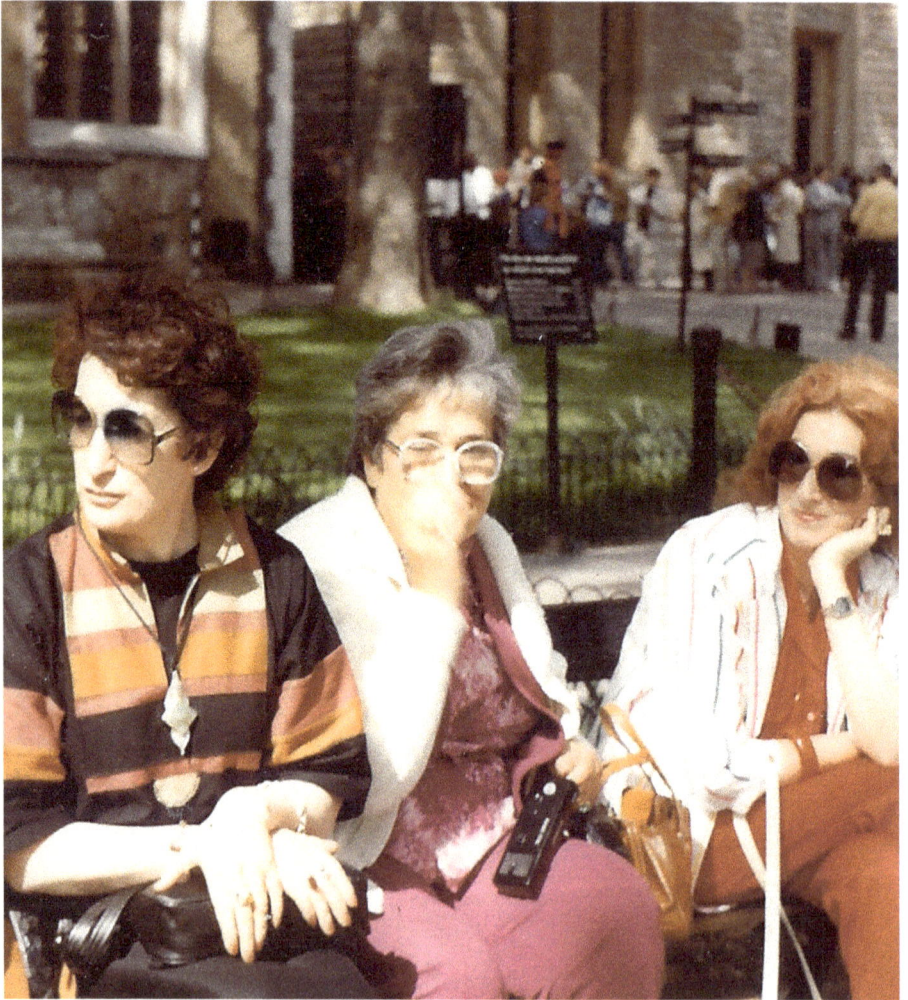

Meeting up with Thelma, mums sister (right) who had flown in to London from the States, with her best friend Ruthy. 1984

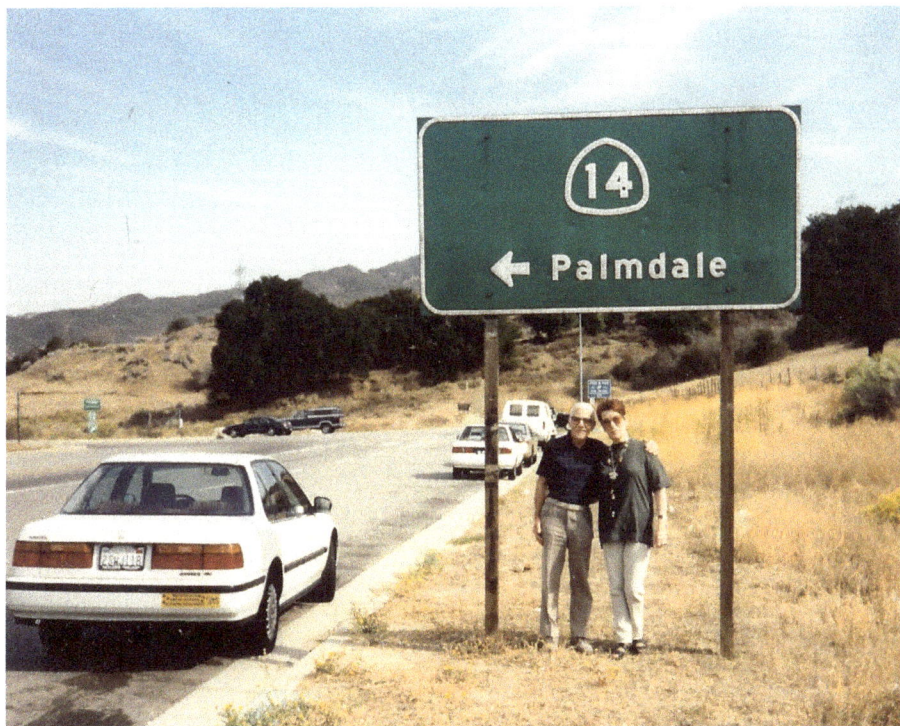

Angela's sister died, but Sam and Angela flew to the States staying with her niece, in Los Angeles.

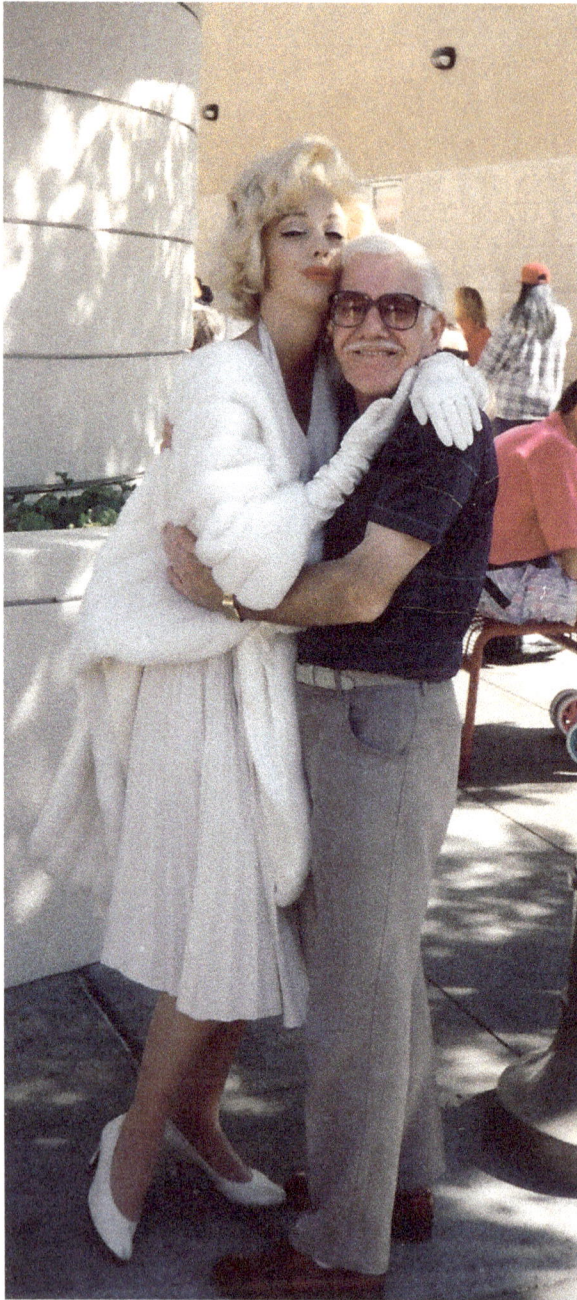

Sam cuddles Marilyn Munroe at Hollywood Studios. Photo taken by Angela 1998.

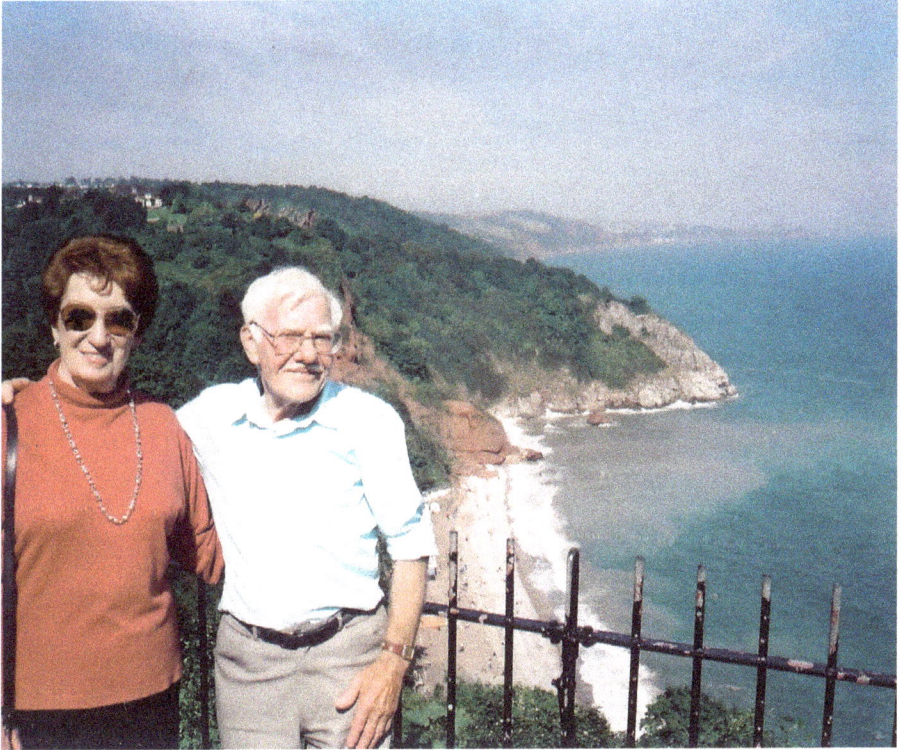

Phil takes Angela and Sam on a touring holiday of the English Riviera during the millenium. Paignton Zoo was a big hit.

Chapter 3:

Role Reversal:
Becoming My Mother's Keeper

L ate autumn light slanted through the kitchen window as my mother stood at the sink, scissors glinting in her hand as she trimmed Mrs. Fenton's hair. Even in her mid-sixties, Angela maintained this small connection to her past work—a few loyal clients who'd become friends over decades, still coming to her home for a cut and conversation. I watched from the doorway, struck by the practiced grace of her movements, unaware that this familiar scene belonged to a chapter of our lives that was rapidly closing.

The first signs appeared with subtle shifts—a wince when she reached for something, her fingers lingering a moment too long on the banister. Then came that afternoon in 2008 when I dropped by after my shift at Cambridge News. She was sitting at the kitchen table, a letter from her doctor spread before her. The news it contained was a sudden and stark reminder of the impending role reversal.

"I've got a double whammy," she said, attempting her usual brightness. "Osteoporosis and rheumatoid arthritis"

I settled into the chair opposite her, processing the words.

"The doctor says I can't go swimming anymore," she added, her disappointment palpable.

"What! But you love swimming?" I protested.

"He's worried if I fall, I'll break something and never recover."

I felt a flare of indignation on her behalf. Swimming had been one of her joys, a freedom she'd maintained even as other activities had gradually fallen away. The prescription seemed wrong—isolating her from something that brought both physical benefit and happiness. This moment marked the first of many medical decisions I would question in the years to come.

Meanwhile, my father's health was deteriorating in less visible ways. Always the stoic ex-army man, he began visiting his doctor with uncharacteristic frequency. His blood pressure had risen, and a strange anxiety had taken hold of him.

One weekend in early 2009, as I sat with him after Sunday lunch—a roast he'd prepared himself—he reached into his pocket and handed me a folded piece of notepaper.

"The doctor wrote this for me," he said.

I unfolded it to find a statement signed by his GP confirming my father's good health. Looking up, I found him watching my reaction intently.

"He says I'm perfectly fit," my father explained. "That I'll go on living for quite some time yet." His determination to live was palpable, a testament to his resilience in the face of uncertainty.

"Why did you ask him for this?" I questioned.

"I told him I didn't think I had long to live."

The paper trembled slightly in my hand. This wasn't the father I knew—the practical engineer who approached problems with methodical logic. Something fundamental had shifted.

A few weeks later, he developed excruciating pain in his leg. I drove him to the surgery, where the doctor, concerned about a possible blood clot, referred us immediately to Addenbrooke's Hospital. The scan revealed not thrombosis but a Baker's cyst. The young nurse using the handheld scanner seemed almost dismissive.

"It's not a blood clot. It's something called a Baker's cyst, which is very similar. Just go home and take painkillers—it will resolve on its own."

We returned home, relieved it wasn't serious, yet unsettled by his continuing discomfort. My father carried on looking after my mother, his own health concerns subordinated to her increasing needs.

While attending art college to complete an access course for university that spring, my phone vibrated during class. My father's voice on the line made no sense—a stream of disconnected words and phrases. Asking to be excused, I rushed home to find him clearly unwell.

The following hours unfold in my memory like a poorly edited film—fragments of police officers in our living room, paramedics taking vitals, and a doctor sitting with my father. Despite my insistence that something was seriously wrong, they left him at home with a prescription rather than admitting him to hospital.

A week later, I found him coughing blood into a handkerchief. This time, my demands couldn't be ignored. He was admitted to Addenbrooke's, where the doctor diagnosed pneumonia with reassuring confidence.

"We can cure that. He should be home in no time."

But the hospital ward didn't match this optimism. It resembled a wartime medical center—understaffed and overwhelmed. My father sat on the edge of a bed while a nursing assistant handed him tissues to catch the blood he continued to cough up. When I questioned the clinician overseeing the ward, she deflected, saying she was still assessing him among many patients.

My voice rising with frustration, I declared, "My father is not going home today."

I left to gather his pajamas and toiletries, determined that he would receive proper care. The following evening, when Angela and I visited, we found a different atmosphere. A nurse approached cheerfully.

"He's been talking to everyone," she said, smiling. "Telling them all about his life."

Yet when *we* sat with him, he was quiet, occasionally reaching for an oxygen mask. The disconnect between the nurse's description and the man before us was jarring.

Returning the following night, I was met by the same nurse, now laughing as she told me, "Your father chewed through the tubes through the night. We found him this morning —".

Her amusement at what was my father's confused behavior felt cruel. I couldn't share in her inappropriate humor as I sat with my increasingly unresponsive father.

On the fourth evening, an auxillary nurse telephoned "Your father, he's not good. Come quick. He's going."

Angela and I hadn't planned to visit that evening, facing the impossible choice of leaving her alone or rushing to his bedside, I gathered my coat and keys, but the phone rang again. He was gone.

I sank into a chair, staring at my mother, who sat like a rabbit caught in headlights—blank, unresponsive, and unable to process the information. The date—October 30, 2009—marked not just my father's passing but the beginning of my new role as my mother's primary caretaker.

Christmas followed and found us at the Royal Cambridge Hotel—my attempt to create normalcy amidst grief. Despite snow covering the grounds on New Year's Day, we drove to Wimpole Hall. Angela had always loved National Trust properties; the grand architecture and carefully preserved rooms gave her a sense of continuity in a world that had suddenly shifted beneath her feet.

I made the difficult decision to abandon my college course, sacrificing once again the university education I'd been working toward. The irony wasn't lost on me—just as a careers advisor had once directed me away from sign writing, circumstances now forced me from art and design. Two paths to creative fulfillment, both closed by forces beyond my control.

By 2012, it became clear that the family home was no longer suitable. The stairs presented an increasing challenge, and I worried constantly about falls. I found a ground-floor retirement flat at Havenfields, not far from Kings Hedges Road. When I showed it to my mother, her initial resistance —"I'm not going into a granny flat"—gave way to

51

appreciation for the thoughtfully furnished space with French doors opening onto communal gardens.

The neighborhood had transformed completely since the 1960s. What had once been fields and woods where I'd played as a child had now been developed into estates, shopping centers, and bypass. The landscape of our shared history had been rewritten, mirroring the changes in our relationship.

Mother's dementia revealed itself in subtle ways at first—repeating questions, staring into the distance with an expression I recognized as deep thought, but which now extended uncomfortably. When she told me, "I don't know what to say," after a visit from her lifelong friend Victor, I recognized the uncharacteristic silence as a warning sign.

Urinary infections became a regular disruption, causing temporary increases in confusion that would clear with antibiotics. Each episode left her slightly diminished.

Yet some joys remained constant. Car rides became her greatest pleasure—sitting in the passenger seat beside me, watching the world race by. Often, she would refuse to exit the vehicle upon our return, preferring to remain seated and observe the street through the windshield. I sometimes left her there briefly, understanding her need to be outside the confines of walls that increasingly defined her existence.

Through these challenging transitions, I found unexpected support. My church community offered practical help and emotional sustenance. Friends invited us for Sunday dinners after services, creating a space where I could temporarily set down the weight of caregiving. These moments of normalcy became essential anchors in a life increasingly defined by medical appointments, medication schedules, and watchful vigils

The reversal of our roles happened not in a single dramatic moment but through countless small surrenders and assumptions of responsibility. The mother who had once chased after me as I played on college punts now depended on me to guide her safely through each day. The woman who had taught me the names of flowers and trees now needed me to interpret the world for her as it grew increasingly confusing.

In becoming my mother's keeper, I discovered capabilities I hadn't known I possessed—patience, tenderness, and advocacy. The boy who had been the focus of Angela's considerable energy and attention was now the man channeling his energy into her care. The circle had closed, not with symmetry or fairness, but with the imperfect beauty of human connection across a lifetime.

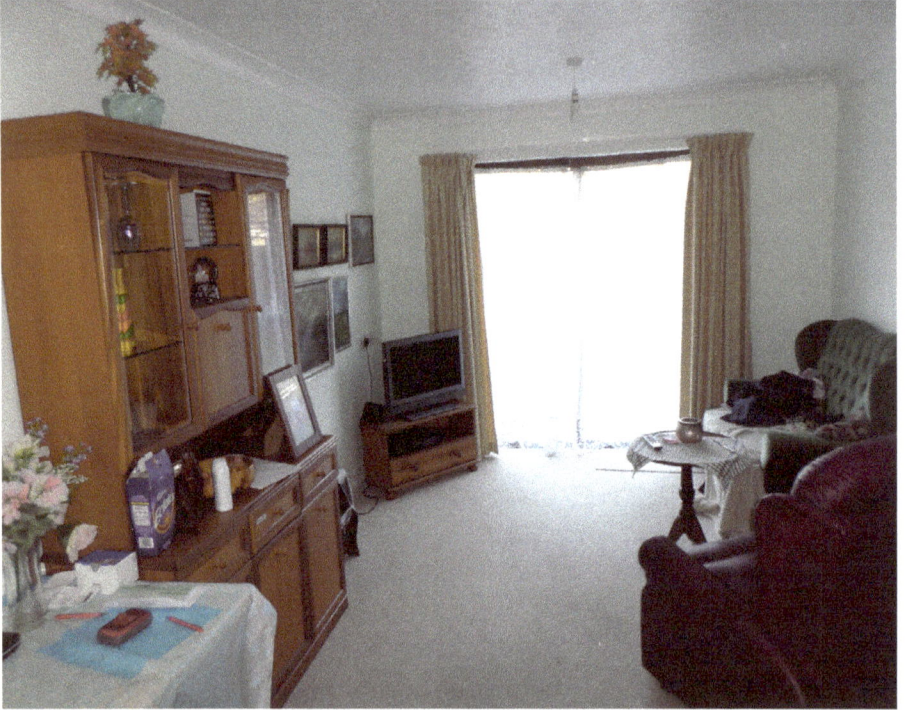

Angel's New flat. 2012.

Chapter 4:

The Hospital Battle Begins

The hospital corridor stretched before me like a battlefield, its institutional lighting casting everything in a harsh, unforgiving glow. Christmas decorations hung limply from the nursing station, their festive intention at odds with the clinical surroundings. I navigated between beds and monitoring equipment, searching for my mother among the rows of elderly patients. December 2014 had already claimed its sacrifices to winter's chill – pneumonia, falls, strokes – and now my mother had joined their ranks.

What I didn't understand then, as I located her bed and pulled a plastic chair close, was that we were crossing a threshold. This wasn't simply another hospital admission; it was the beginning of a systematic separation. The battle for her future was already being planned in meeting rooms I wasn't invited to enter.

My phone rang three days after her admission. The voice was professional, detached.

"Mr. Webb? I'm calling from the Clinical Commissioning Group regarding your mother, Angela Webb."

I listened as the caller explained their role in "transitioning" patients from hospital to "appropriate ongoing care." The carefully selected terminology masked what they were really saying: my mother wouldn't be coming home.

"We believe your mother requires continued hospital-level care," the voice informed me. "This can best be provided in a specialized facility."

No questions about how I'd managed her care for years. No acknowledgment of our established routines and systems. Just a clinical assessment made by strangers who had known her for days rather than decades.

"Do you have power of attorney?" they asked.

I did – for financial matters – but I soon learned this wasn't enough. Without lasting power of attorney for health and welfare, my ability to challenge their decisions was severely limited. A bureaucratic detail would determine the course of our lives.

Within days, they'd identified a bed at Buchen House care home. Angela was transported there by ambulance, the transition executed with efficient detachment. When I arrived to see her settled in this new environment, the manager approached with papers outlining the costs: nearly £4,000 monthly – a staggering £1,000 per week.

"But the hospital arranged this," I protested. "Surely they cover the costs?"

The uncomfortable pause that followed confirmed my naivety. After assessment, the authorities contributed between five and ten percent of the fees – a token gesture that did little to address the financial chasm opening before me. The remainder would come from my mother's savings, the nest egg she and my father had carefully built over decades.

As I visited Buchen House daily, I watched winter turn to spring through the windows. Angela's room became familiar

—the institutional bed with its adjustable rails, the laminate bedside table, and the chair where I sat for hours. Six months passed this way, a holding pattern that drained both her savings and my resolve.

As summer approached, I made my decision. The care home had failed to improve her condition; in fact, she seemed diminished – less mobile, less engaged. I decided to bring her home to her Havenfield flat, despite what anyone else may think.

I knew something they didn't: the woman being kept in bed for twenty hours a day was the same woman who had once chased me across college grounds, who had joined the boys in their neighborhood games. Beneath the frailty lay resilience I was determined to reawaken.

The day I brought her home, the simple joy on her face as she entered her own space confirmed my decision. I spent the following weeks rigorously attending to her needs while simultaneously tackling the overwhelming task of decluttering her Kings Hedges Road house. The physical labor of sorting through decades of family possessions provided a counterpoint to the delicate work of helping my mother regain strength.

Our victory was short-lived. On March 10, 2016, Angela fell again. The familiar ambulance journey to Addenbrooke's replayed like a recurring nightmare. This time, however, the hospital's assessment surprised me.

"She can walk more than five meters with a frame," the discharge nurse reported on March 14. "She's ready to return home."

This unexpected reprieve came with community support – a nurse who visited fortnightly, bringing practical solutions like sliding sheets that made transferring Angela from bed to wheelchair smoother and safer. The system, it seemed, could work with us rather than against us.

Through spring and summer, we established a routine. I wheeled her through the French doors of her ground-floor flat, allowing her to enjoy the communal gardens. The birds at the feeder outside her window became companions, squirrels performing acrobatics on the lawn provided entertainment. Small pleasures accumulated, creating a life that, while limited, contained dignity and moments of joy.

Then August 28, 2016, arrived. Another fall, another ambulance, another admission to Addenbrooke's. But something had changed in the ward's atmosphere. Staff exchanged glances when I visited, their eyes following me with an assessment that had nothing to do with medical care.

During one visit, a woman in a dark blue uniform—not the pale blue of regular nurses—approached me. Her uniform signaled authority, and her clipboard a shield.

"Mr. Webb, we need to discuss your mother's financial situation," she began without preamble.

"I'm here to discuss her health," I countered.

"The two are connected," she persisted. "How much money does your mother have?"

The bluntness of the question shocked me. This wasn't about Angela's wellbeing; it was an audit of resources, an assessment of worth based on financial metrics rather than human needs. I refused to answer, feeling blood rising to my face.

In the following days, I was required to complete questionnaires that reduced my mother's existence to numerical scores. Can she feed herself? Rate from zero to ten. Can she communicate effectively? Another number. Can she maintain continence? Each question carried hidden weight, determining whether she would qualify for funding in care.

The results, when they came, were predictable. Angela scored too well for full funding but poorly enough to require institutional care—the worst possible combination. As consolation, a "discretionary payment" amounting to about five percent of costs was offered.

A social worker suddenly materialized next, clipboard in hand and sympathetic smile firmly in place.

"This is a list of all care homes in Cambridgeshire," she explained, handing me several densely printed pages. "You need to choose one."

I stared at the document – nearly 200 facilities listed with minimal information about each.

"How long do I have?" I asked.

"We need a decision quickly," she replied, the smile never wavering. "The hospital needs the bed."

The impossibility of the task overwhelmed me. How could I assess 200 unfamiliar places with their own approaches, atmospheres, and standards? How could I determine which might provide genuine care rather than mere containment?

Buchan House, where Angela had previously stayed, was no longer an option. The manager remembered the missed transport incident and refused to accommodate her again. The Hollies, another facility where she had briefly been happy, had closed down – financial casualties of actually providing quality care.

In desperation, I selected Midfield Lodge in Oakington based on location and availability rather than any meaningful criteria. The former young offenders' facility retained its institutional character – rectangular corridors surrounding a central courtyard, reminiscent of a prison exercise yard. When I first visited, Angela had been placed in a room with blank walls and no view, compounding her disorientation and distress.

After persistent requests, they moved her to a room with views of fields and trees. It was a small victory in a war I was clearly losing – the ability to make fundamental decisions about my mother's care was being systematically removed from my hands.

The transfer to Midfield Lodge occurred in October 2016. I watched as hospital transport delivered my mother to yet another unfamiliar environment, her belongings in a small bag, her confusion evident. She would now sleep in a room she hadn't chosen, be cared for by strangers whose names she couldn't remember, and follow routines established for institutional efficiency rather than individual comfort.

As I left that first evening, walking down the corridor that echoed with distant televisions and occasional calls for assistance, the magnitude of what was happening crystallized. This wasn't simply a medical decision or a matter of practical care; it was a fundamental question of autonomy and dignity.

Who had the right to determine how Angela would spend her remaining years? Who truly understood her needs, preferences, and the small details that made life worth living?

The system had provided an answer I couldn't accept. The healthcare machinery had assessed, processed, and allocated my mother according to protocols and available resources. But their calculations had overlooked something crucial – the immeasurable value of family care, familiarity, and being surrounded by the small comforts of home.

I stepped out into the autumn evening, keys gripped tightly in my hand. The battle had shifted now. No longer was I simply advocating for appropriate medical care; I was fighting for my mother's right to live her final years with dignity, in surroundings of her choosing, cared for by those who truly knew her.

The hospital phase might have ended, but the war was just beginning. As I drove away from Midfield Lodge that evening, leaving my mother in her new room with its majetic view of a carpark, I made a silent promise: this would not be the end of our story.

Chapter 5:

Life In Limbo:
The Care Home Years

T he autumn wind swept across the fields surrounding Midfield Lodge as I approached the entrance for my daily visit. I arrived with the copper-colored leaves and a growing sense of permanence about my mother's situation. Each visit required a deliberate mental preparation—steeling myself against the institutional smells, the sound of distant televisions blaring at excessive volume, and the sight of my mother confined to an environment neither of us had chosen.

Midfield Lodge retained the unmistakable architecture of its previous incarnation as a young offenders' facility. Four connected corridors formed a rectangle around a central courtyard, creating a layout that felt more designed for containment than comfort. My footsteps echoed against the linoleum as I made my way to my mother's room, nodding to staff members who had begun to recognize my daily appearances.

The rhythms of institutional care gradually emerged through my observations. Some days, I would arrive to find Angela animated, having spoken with carers and other residents. Sebastian, the nursing officer, would approach with updates: "She's been chatting away this morning." On other days, she retreated into profound silence as though withdrawing from a world that had become increasingly incomprehensible. This inconsistency—these glimpses of my mother's true self followed by prolonged absences—became a particular kind of torture.

During one visit, I noticed my mother shifting uncomfortably in bed. When I investigated the cause, I discovered the beginning of bedsore—an angry red mark that signaled sustained pressure and inadequate movement.

"This shouldn't be happening," I told Lee Jay, the head nurse and deputy manager.

"It's nothing to worry about," he assured me. "We can heal it. We can get it cured."

But the practical follow-through didn't match his confidence. The care home used special pressure-relief mattresses—rubber lilos that constantly moved to prevent pressure points. I questioned their effectiveness in bringing in a comfortable foam mattress topper I'd purchased.

When he discovered my attempt, Lee Jay said firmly, "You can't have that on top. That will restrict how the mattress works."

Mother's voice suddenly interrupted as we debated this: "What's that up there?"

We both turned to see her pointing toward the corner of the ceiling. "Up there, look," she insisted, eyes fixed on something invisible to us.

Lee Jay gave me a knowing look. "This is what happens," he said quietly as we left the room. "It's part of the end-of-life process."

But I knew my mother. This wasn't the first time she had seemed to hallucinate. When she had urinary tract infections in the past, similar episodes had occurred. I bypassed Lee Jay and called her doctor directly.

The bedsore wasn't the mother's only physical concern. Open wounds had developed on her feet, particularly her toes. Eventually, I secured an appointment with a specialist at Addenbrooke's. After examining her, he delivered unexpected good news.

"Your mother has circulation going to her feet, which is positive," he explained. "These wounds can heal if she exercises. Have her move her ankles and toes regularly."

Following his instructions, I began daily exercises with Angela encouraging her to flex her feet and wiggle her toes. "If you don't do this, you could lose your feet," I told her plainly. Remarkably, she understood and cooperated. Over time, the wounds began to heal—a vindication of my instinct that proper attention could improve her condition rather than merely manage her decline.

Food became another battleground. The care home served mother's meals completely mashed together—meat, vegetables, and potatoes transformed into an unidentifiable orange mush that resembled blancmange more than dinner. No wonder she wasn't eating. She couldn't even have her preferred breakfast of Cornflakes or Rice Krispies, it had to be porridge, 'but it was formely an offenders institution,' but I didn't find that thought funny.

After witnessing this, I approached the staff about feeding her properly.

"If you want to give her solid food, you'll need to sign a declaration," Lee Jay informed me. "You'll be responsible if anything happens."

I signed immediately, then began arriving at mealtimes to feed her myself. We operated outside the rigid timetables of institutional care. While other residents were hurried through meals so staff could clear tables and move to the next task, Angela and I existed in our own time zone. I cut her food into small, appetizing pieces, feeding her slowly and patiently. Often, we were the first to arrive in the dining room and the last to leave, sometimes two hours later.

Within this regimented environment, I sought allies. Sebastian, the head nurse, showed genuine compassion. Sue Cox, one of the regular carers, developed a special relationship with my mother, taking extra time with her. Even Lee Jay, despite our disagreements, occasionally provided helpful information. During one of our conversations, he mentioned something that lodged in my mind.

"Your mother is a private patient," he said. "You're paying for her. You can take her home if you want."

This matter of fact contradicted everything social services told me. I filed this information away, sensing its potential importance.

Then came the day I noticed my mother's rings were missing—her wedding ring and eternity ring with a one-and-a-half-carat diamond in eighteen-carat gold, gifts from my father that she had worn for decades. I alerted the staff immediately, setting off a frantic search of her room, bed linens, and the shower area. Nothing.

The police were called, and what followed was a strange subplot in our ongoing drama. A Hungarian agency worker approached me privately, smiling as he wrote down the name of a female colleague he claimed had taken the rings. Later, when the investigating officer interviewed this woman, she laughed and explained the accusation was revenge for her rejecting the Hungarian worker's romantic advances. The investigation stalled when, on the day police interviewed staff, only agency workers were present—none of the regular staff who knew about the rings were scheduled.

"The manager chose a day when we weren't there," one regular staff member later told me. "We were the ones who knew your mom and her rings."

The case was eventually closed without resolution—another small indignity in a mounting collection of losses.

As weeks turned to months, I developed parallel support networks. The Dixons and the Newmans, friends from church, provided regular dinners and conversation—spaces where I could momentarily set down the weight of constant advocacy. A Bible study group in Burwell offered spiritual sustenance. Most practically, I joined a carers' support group where I met Ted, a remarkable man in his nineties who was successfully caring for his wife at home.

Ted became an unlikely mentor. "There's nothing to stop you from taking your mum out of there," he said when I explained my frustrations. Despite his age—or perhaps because of it—he possessed clarity about navigating the system that younger people lacked.

Through church connections, I encountered the Hertfordshire Adult Social Services manager, who advised me to write letters to the council and social services explaining my intentions. These strategic relationships provided emotional support and practical intelligence about the system I was battling.

Institutional resistance manifested in a series of confrontational meetings. During one session with a social worker regarding my mother's health issues, I found myself facing complete dismissal.

When I raised concerns, she stated bluntly, "I don't care what you say. Your mother is staying here."

I stood up, unable to contain my frustration. "You don't know what you're talking about," I responded. "You don't know my mother and certainly don't know me."

This encounter led to a second meeting with the social worker's supervisor and an advocate I'd arranged to accompany me. The tone shifted noticeably with this additional support. The supervisor actually discussed the possibility of my mother leaving the facility, suggesting we could transition her to a care home closer to where I wanted to live. I left feeling I'd crossed "halfway to where I wanted to be"—a small victory in an ongoing campaign.

Through conversations with staff and research, I made a crucial discovery: the care home lacked a "deprivation of liberty" order for my mother. This legal document would have been necessary to keep her incarcerated against my wishes. The absence of this order created a potential opening.

I began testing the system's boundaries by taking my mother out for short visits. Initially, I asked permission to bring her back to her flat for a few hours. The staff, seeing nothing unusual in a son wanting time with his mother, readily agreed. Each successful outing built my confidence and provided valuable information about my mother's tolerance for travel and change.

During these excursions, a transformation occurred. Angela who often sat silently in her care home room would become animated once in the taxi, gazing out with evident pleasure. When we arrived at her flat, she recognized her surroundings and relaxed visibly. These responses strengthened my conviction that the institutional setting was diminishing rather than supporting her.

While spending time at my mother's flat during these visits, I began methodically preparing it for her potential return— cleaning thoroughly, adjusting furniture for wheelchair access, and investigating equipment I might need. These preparations were partly practical and partly an act of faith— a physical manifestation of my refusal to accept the current situation as permanent.

The hardest moments came when returning mother to Midfield Lodge. As we approached the building, her expression would change, a subtle shutdown occurring as we reentered the institutional environment. Signing her back in felt like a betrayal each time, a temporary surrender in a war I was determined to ultimately win.

Winter turned to spring, then summer. My daily visits continued, each one reinforcing the disconnect between the care I knew my mother deserved and what institutional limitations allowed. I watched residents move efficiently through daily routines—bathing, meals, medication—with minimal regard for individual preferences or identities. The system wasn't cruel; it was designed for processing rather than nurturing.

On Sunday afternoons, I sometimes sat in church, not hearing the sermon but contemplating the nature of family obligation and love. What did it mean to honor my mother in these circumstances? Was acceptance of expert opinions the right path, or was resistance the true expression of filial duty? My home group Bible study leader at Burwell, knowing I wanted mum home asked directly,

"What's holding you back, Philip?" "You seem to lack confidence when confronting authority."

His observation cut through months of hesitation, this in conjuction with Joel Dixon's offer to help me bust her out of there, was the catalist I needed to put thought into action. The group prayed for me, and something crystallized in that moment of community support. The question wasn't whether I could challenge the system but whether I could live with myself if I didn't try.

As autumn 2017 approached, marking nearly a year at Midfield Lodge, I moved from contemplation to planning. The daily visits, the accumulation of knowledge about my mother's care, the network of supporters, and the legal research all converged toward a single point of action. In quiet moments between institutional routines, I began forming a plan that many would call impossible—a plan to bring my mother home.

The limbo of care home existence—neither fully living nor actively dying—had persisted too long. As I left Midfield Lodge one evening, as I passed mums window towards the carpark, I saw her looking up at the tall trees oppersite an I made my decision. The next phase would require courage, thinig, and a willingness to risk everything for the simple belief that a mother deserved to be cared for by the son she had once cared for so completely.

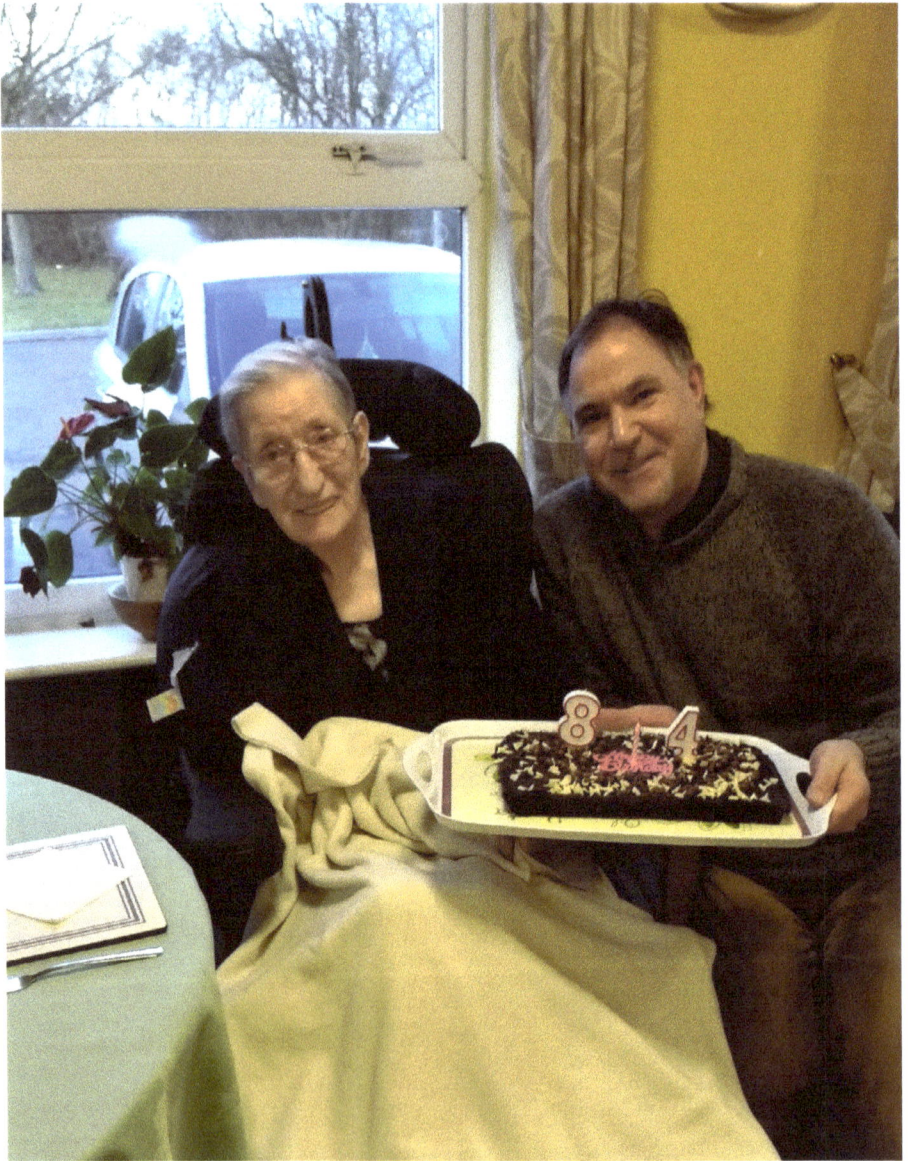

"We just have to make the best of it, its all we can do now". Mum is presented with a birthdaycake at Midfield Lodge.

Chapter 6:

Planning The Great Escape

January winds cut across Kessingland beach with surgical precision as I walked alone, my footsteps disappearing in the pebbles behind me. The winter solitude had drawn me here—Angela, warm in the carehome and safe —providing a rare moment to breathe without the weight of constant vigilance. I trod further, the crunching stones beneath my feet creating the only sound for miles.

The beach stretched empty before me, a liminal space between decisions. Mother had been in the care home since October, and with each passing day, the institutional machinery tightened its grip. The financial drain was becoming unsustainable, her savings diminishing while her spirit faded under fluorescent lights and regulated routines.

I stopped where the land curved toward the horizon. No other human figure interrupted the vast emptiness of sky meeting sea. Something shifted in this moment of absolute solitude—a clarity descending as tangible as the January air.

"This is where I should start looking," I heard myself say aloud, the words carried away on the wind.

The thought hadn't been there a moment before, yet now it stood fully formed: I needed to move away from Cambridge, from the jurisdiction of those who had taken control of mother's care. Suffolk, with its coastal towns and different administrative boundaries, offered possibility.

From that beach, I drove directly into Lowestoft, walked into an estate agent's office, and found and secured a house within two weeks. The speed of events felt supernatural, as though forces beyond myself were orchestrating what logic said was impossible.

Practical matters followed with the same uncanny momentum. The mortgage broker barely blinked at my circumstances, approving £130,000 based on my flat as collateral. Mother's investment fund provided the £30,000 deposit. Financial pieces aligned with suspicious ease, as though the universe itself conspired to clear obstacles.

"The house has nothing in it," I explained to a removal company based in Lowestoft. "But I need to bring furniture from two properties in Cambridge."

They agreed to collect selected items from my mother's house and retirement flat. I marked out key pieces—her display cabinet, paitings, ornamentals that carried anchors of familiarity I would need to recreate her world.

The bedroom presented particular challenges. Angela had become increasingly immobile in the care home, kept in bed for long periods that diminished her strength. I searched online auction sites, eventually purchasing an adjustable hospital bed with side rails—the kind with remote controls that could raise her to a sitting position or elevate her feet as needed.

Equipment research consumed my evenings. The most critical piece would be a means of transferring mother between the wheelchair and the car. The care home insisted such transfers required two trained staff—a requirement designed to make independent care seem impossible. I refused to accept this as truth.

Late one night, scrolling through disability equipment sites, I discovered the Milford car-to-wheelchair transfer system— an ingenious hoist that's welded permanently to a car's chassis allowing a single person to safely transfer someone from wheelchair to passenger seat. The new models cost thousands, well beyond my means.

Further research led me to a garden center that sold refurbished disability equipment. They listed a Milford Mark 2 S25 system at approximately one-third of the retail price. When I called, the seller proved unexpectedly helpful.

"Do you know how to fit one of these?" he asked after I'd confirmed my interest.

"Absolutely not," I admitted.

"They're quite complex. You can't just bolt them in—they need proper installation to be safe," he explained. "I know someone in Mansfield who specializes in mobility equipment installation. I could send it directly to him, save you the delivery charge, and you could arrange a fitting with him."

Another piece fell into place.

November 7th arrived—the day scheduled for this hoist installation. I woke at 5:00 AM to drive to Mansfield, drawing back the curtains to a scene from mythology. Rain wasn't just falling, it was hurtling down with perfect perpendicular precision, so heavy that the audible impact was distracting and unsettling. The sky was a solid dark mass from horizon to horizon.

As I stood watching this deluge, doubt crept in. Was this a sign? The biblical scale of the downpour seemed deliberately placed to test my resolve. For a moment, I hesitated.

Gathering my resolve, saying "Wild horses cannot stop me now."

The journey proved treacherous. Windscreen wipers struggled against the torrent, and standing water gathered on motorways. I passed three accidents before reaching my exit from the A1. Yet, as arranged, I arrived precisely at 8:15 AM.

The installer and his young apprentice greeted me.

"This will take all day," he warned. "We'll need to remove the seats and take up the floor. It's quite involved."

I wandered Mansfield through the continuing rain, playing tourist in a city I'd never visited. I deliberately turned my phone off to immerse myself in the anonymity of exploration. When I returned at 5:00 PM, the installer's expression suggested complication.

"We've been trying to reach you," he began. "When we removed the floor, your car was full of water. We tried ringing you to cancel but we couldnt get hold of you. We dried it out as best we could and completed the installation."

He demonstrated the system, showing me how the components slotted together, how the remote control raised and lowered the arm, and how the safety harness attached. Despite the water issue, his work was immaculate.

Driving back toward Cambridge that evening, I felt a piece of armor slide into place. One determined son could now accomplish the impossible, to bust her out of there without anyone knowing how!

The car hoist solved one crucial problem, but another hoist would also be necessary. Through another online search, I located a secondhand portable room hoist in Walton-on-the-Naze, still under warranty. The following day, I drove there to meet the owner who had only just become a widower.

"She's only been gone two months," he explained as he demonstrated the hoist's operation. "It was serviced just before..."

He didn't need to finish the sentence, I nodded understandly.

With both hoists secured, I turned to the administrative groundwork—the paper trail that would need to disappear behind us. My mother's medical records presented the first challenge. If questions arose after her removal, authorities would immediately contact her GP.

So I visited the surgery appointed by the care home, approaching the receptionist with casual confidence.

"I need to change my mother's doctor," I stated. "She's moving to a different area."

No questions were asked. Mum's records were transferred to a practice near Havenfields—a temporary measure before their final transfer to a Lowestoft surgery. This created a paper trail that would lead away from, rather than toward, our actual destination.

Strategic help would be essential. Munaza, the tenant in mother's house, had become a trusted ally since moving in. Over drinks, after watching the movie "Bohemian Rhapsody" at the cinema one evening, I carefully outlined the operation.

"I don't want to say too much in case someone in authority comes asking questions," I explained, "but I'm going to take my mother out of the care home."

"When?" she asked simply.

"This week, if you can help. Are you free the sixteenth through eighteenth?"

She nodded. "What do you need me to do?"

I explained that after I'd removed my mother, Munaza would need to go to Midfield Lodge and clear her room—all personal items, nothing was to remain. She would then hand a letter I'd written to the staff then drive staight to Lowestoft.

"If they ask what you're doing, just say 'Philip wants everything out' and hand them the letter as you leave."

In the meantime I arranged for my son Austin to visit his grandmother at the care home, I wanted him to see her one last time in case the worst happened, or legalalities prevented future contact.

Their last afternoon together was important—Austin sat beside his grandmother as camera's clicked. The visit provided—a normal family connection raising no suspicions among staff, except I knew that would be the last time Austin would see his grandmother.

In Angela's bedroom at Havenfield, I composed the letter that would formalize our departure. It stated simply that I was removing my mother from the care home and taking her

THE GREAT ESCAPE LOVE DUTY AND DEFIANCE

home, Midfield Lodge lacked any legal authority to prevent this, having no deprivation of liberty in place, there was nothing they could do. I then sealed it and gave it to Munaza and drove to Lowestoft.

The night before my departure, I prepared Mum's bedroom in Lowestoft one final time. The bed was in position, the hoist stood ready beside it, wardrobe, chest of drawers, space for tv, everything necessary for her care was in place.

I drove back to Cambridge, arriving late. Sleep proved elusive as I mentally rehearsed each step of tomorrow's operation. The car journey would take approximately two hours. The transfer from wheelchair to car seat using the Milford hoist would be the most challenging moment—it had to be executed smoothly, rapidly, and away from prying eyes.

Like any military planner, I had identified the vulnerabilities in my operation. If the staff at Midfield Lodge suspected anything, they might refuse to have Angela ready. If the taxi driver realized what was happening, he might report back. If my mother became distressed during the journey, complications could multiply.

Yet beneath these tactical concerns lay a deeper certainty —this was right. The system that had taken control of my mother's care had failed her. The bedsores, the foot wounds, the institutional food, and the stolen rings all testified to a fundamental truth: she belonged with me, not in a facility designed for processing rather than nurturing.

As dawn approached, I finally drifted into a shallow sleep, dreaming of corridors that led nowhere and doors that wouldn't open. When the alarm sounded at 6:00 AM, I rose with the calm that comes after a decision has replaced deliberation.

Today, we would go home—not to Havenfield where the system could easily find us, not to the house where memories of my father lingered, but to a new beginning in Lowestoft, where the sea air carried possibilities rather than restrictions.

In a few hours, if all went well, we would cross an administrative boundary providing at least temporary protection from those who believed they knew better than a son his mother needed.

Walking to my car, keys in hand, I felt a peculiar lightness. The morning air seemed charged with potential. Whatever happened next—success or failure, freedom or consequences—I had chosen action over acceptance which would lay the outcome of the day.

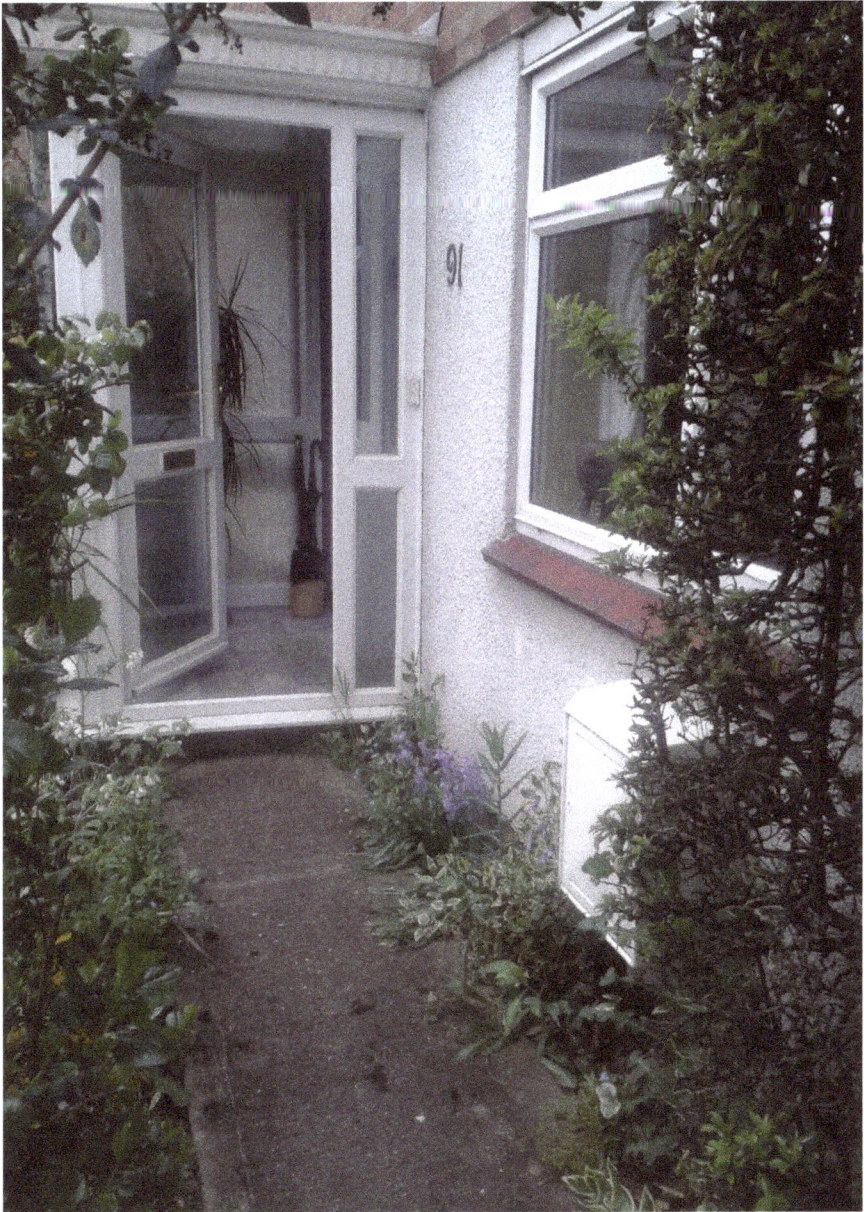

Staying at 91 in anticipation of the secret operation, only I knew was about to happen, soon we would be somewhere else.

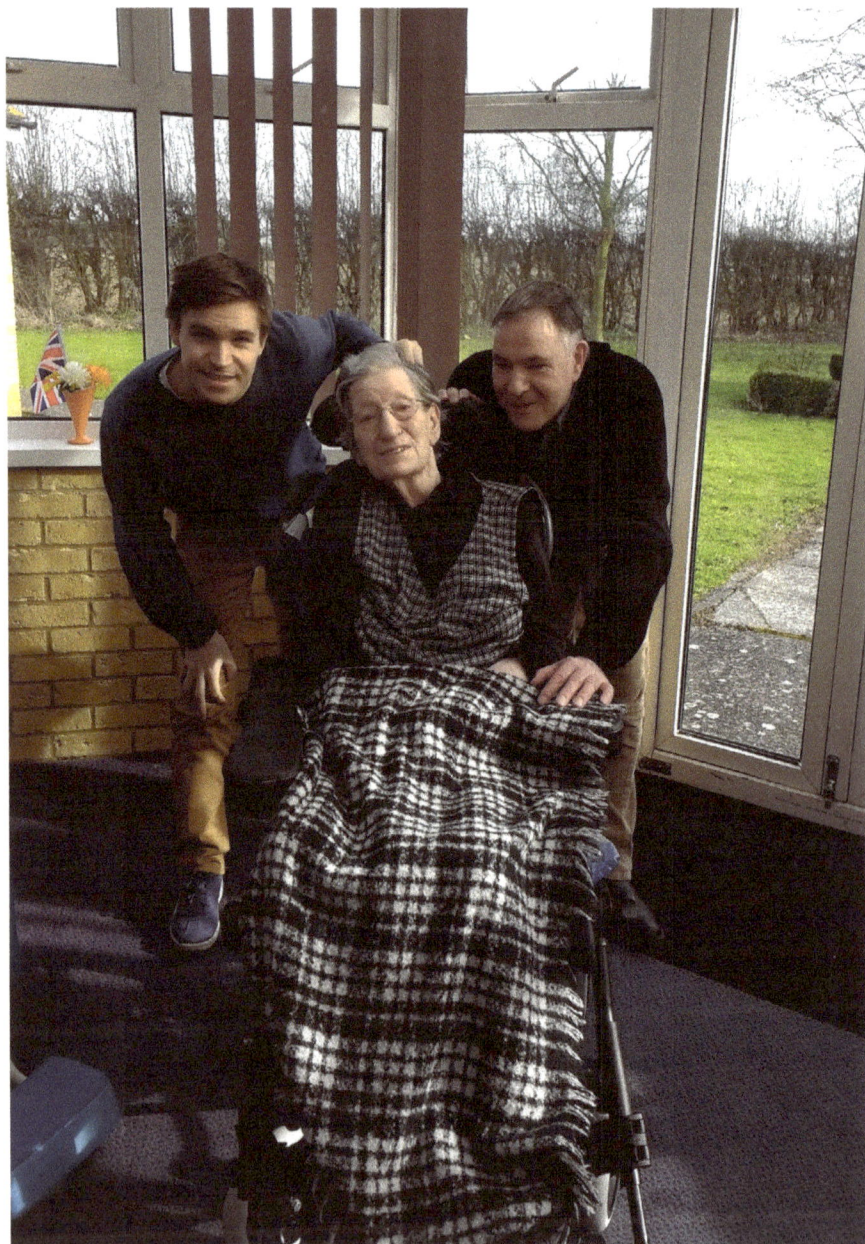

Here are the three of us together for the last time: Austin, Angela's Grandson
and her son Phil,

Chapter 7:

The Day Of Deliverance: November 15th

Dawn broke with surprising gentleness on November 15th. After biblical downpours during my journey to Mansfield for the hoist installation, this Thursday morning offered a stillness that felt almost conspiratorial. I stood at the window of my mother's Havenfield flat, watching early light illuminate a world unaware of what was about to unfold. At 10:30 AM, I carried my overnight bag to the car, positioned the Zafira facing outward for a quick departure, then waited at the front entrance, watching the odd resident beginning their daily chores.

The taxi arrived precisely at 11:00 AM. "Midfield Lodge in Oakington?," I asked in a casual manner, then after taking my seat we were off. Once we arrived I signed the visitors' book as I had hundreds of times, just as a uniformed carer approached, "You're right on time. Your mother's all ready." Angela sat in her wheelchair, dressed in a blue cardigan of some description and white blouse I'd brought months earlier. Her hair brushed, a hint of powder on her cheeks. This small effort at presentation for what staff believed was simply a day trip caught me unexpectedly.

The carer handed me a small bag containing icontinence pads, "when are you bringing her back?" another asked, "er, not sure... but you'll hear from me later," I replied, deliberately ambiguous which passed without comment. The taxi driver wheeled mum into the back of the taxi and I sat in the seat next to her.

Twenty minutes later, we arrived at Havenfields. The driver helped navigate my mother from the taxi to the pavement. I paid him, adding a generous tip.

"I'll call when we need to go back" I said, which wasn't a lie technically, but felt like one.

I waited until his taxi disappeared down the driveway and out of sight—the first phase complete. I turned mother's wheelchair around and pushed it directly to my parked car.

"This is going to be fun, Mum," I said softly, opening the passenger door to reveal the installed hoist system.

Working methodically, I assembled the hoist just as I'd practiced. Mum watched silently, her eyes following my movements with a mixture of curiosity and trust. I carefully fitted the safety harness around her, explaining each step. Her only response was a slight nod, but the absence of resistance spoke volumes.

The mechanism purred softly as it lifted my mother from the wheelchair. I guided the arm, rotating until she was positioned over the passenger seat, then gradually lowered her down. The transfer took about twenty minutes—no drama, just quiet efficiency of well-engineered equipment and careful planning.

"We're off," I said simply as I started the engine. "We're going on a long journey now, Mum."

As we pulled away, I scanned my mirrors constantly, half-expecting a pursuit that never materialized. We reached the

A14 without incident, joining eastbound traffic toward Bury St. Edmunds. At Bury, we turned onto the A143—chosen specifically for its scenic route and fewer roundabouts.

"It's just like old times, isn't it?" I glanced at my mother.

"Yes, it is," she replied, her voice stronger than I'd heard in months. "Keep driving."

Those five words—the most coherent sentence she'd spoken in weeks—validated everything. I gripped the steering wheel tighter, emotion threatening to blur my vision.

We arrived at the Lowestoft house around 2:30 PM. The reverse transfer went even more smoothly than the first. I assembled the car hoist, secured the harness, and lifted her from the seat into the waiting wheelchair. Then I pushed her directly into her prepared bedroom, where the day hoist stood ready.

This final transfer—from wheelchair to bed—completed our journey. I positioned mother comfortably, adjusting pillows and covering her with the duvet I'd selected for its similarity to the one from her flat. The relief on her face as she settled into a non-institutional bed was unmistakable.

With Angela settled in I turned my phone off completely, this moment deserved protection from the outside world.

Meanwhile, the second phase unfolded back in Cambridge. Munaza drove to Midfield Lodge as arranged, collected all mother's possessions, and when questioned by a carer, responded with practiced simplicity: "Philip wants everything out." Only after securing all belongings in her car did she deliver my prepared letter. The manager's realization that Angela wasn't coming back would have been something to witness, but by then, Munaza was gone, our mission quietly completed.

That evening, I became Angela's sole care giver again. She seemed uncomfortable, shifting constantly despite the quality mattress. When I investigated, I discovered the root cause of problems the care home never addressed—severe constipation. No wonder they'd reported her as "off her food" and placed her on palliative care. The issue wasn't appetite but discomfort so severe it made eating unbearable.

What followed was a difficult but necessary intervention that no son imagines performing for a parent. Yet in that moment of intimate care, the boundaries between caregiver and son, between dignity and necessity, dissolved into something more fundamental—the simple human act of relieving suffering.

The relief was immediate and dramatic. By morning, Angela was accepting small amounts of food again—the beginning of a recovery the care home had deemed impossible.

As she drifted to sleep that night, I sat beside her bed, watching the rhythmic rise and fall of her breathing. Outside, the intermittent sound of seagulls provided a gentle soundtrack to our new beginning. We had traversed the gap between institutional care and family love, between professional detachment and personal commitment.

Whatever challenges lay ahead, whatever consequences, we had won something precious—the right to care for family on our own terms, with love rather than institutional efficiency.

We had found our way back home.

Chapter 8:

Standing Our Ground

The November sun rose over Lowestoft with tentative warmth, filtering through unfamiliar curtains into the downstairs bedroom where my mother slept peacefully. One day had passed since our journey from Cambridge—twenty-four hours of freedom from institutional routines and clinical assessments. I moved quietly around the kitchen, preparing tea and toast, stealing occasional glances through the doorway at the rhythmic rise and fall of her breathing.

My phone remained deliberately powered down, tucked into a drawer like a loaded weapon I wasn't yet ready to deploy. Its silence provided a protective bubble around our new beginning, insulating us from the storm I knew was gathering in Cambridge. The house quiet—broken only by the distant call of gulls and the gentle hum of the heating system—felt sacred, a space where healing could begin without interruption.

Angela woke around nine, her eyes briefly registering confusion before recognition settled across her features.

"Good morning," I said, carrying in her tea. "Welcome to your new home."

She accepted the cup with a slight nod, her gaze drifting to the window where winter light played across unfamiliar walls.

We had crossed a threshold together, and now we needed to find our footing in this new territory.

That first week unfolded in a curious mix of ordinary routines and extraordinary vigilance. Each morning, I checked the street before drawing back the curtains, half-expecting to find official vehicles idling at the curb. Each afternoon, I walked to the corner shop for supplies, hurrying back as though my absence might create an opportunity for intervention.

After nearly a week of this self-imposed isolation, I finally retrieved my phone from the drawer. Taking a deep breath, I pressed the power button, bracing myself for the cascade of notifications I knew would follow. The screen lit up, followed immediately by a rapid succession of alert sounds—text messages, voicemails, missed calls accumulating with unsettling speed.

I scrolled through them, categorizing the senders: Cambridgeshire Police, repeating urgent requests to contact them regarding Angela Webb; the head of Cambridgeshire Adult Social Services, demanding immediate communication; Cheryl, the manager of Midfield Lodge, asking me to discuss what was happening. Each message carried the same underlying message: return what you have taken.

Rather than responding directly to these demands, I decided on a more measured approach. I took a photograph of my mother sitting up in bed, smiling with a cup of tea in her hands. The image captured exactly what I wanted to convey —she was comfortable, cared for, and happy. I sent this to

Cheryl at Midfield Lodge with a brief message: "As you can see, my mother is very comfortable. She has all she needs."

Her reply came quickly: "A very nice photograph, Philip, but that's not enough. That won't do it for me. I need more information."

I didn't respond. Instead, I turned my attention to the most pressing authority—the police. Calling the Cambridgeshire Constabulary, I identified myself immediately.

"Mr Webb here. I've received several messages from you regarding my mother."

"Oh yes," the officer replied, "We need to establish your mother's whereabouts."

"She's with me," I stated simply.

"And where is that?"

"In Lowestoft."

There was a pause, followed by papers being shuffled. "So you're not in Cambridge?"

"No, I'm in Suffolk, not in your jurisdiction."

Another pause. "Can you provide her address?"

I did so, sensing the shift in dynamic. The officer's voice lost its edge of urgency. "Leave it with us," he said finally.

Within days, the transfer was complete. Cambridgeshire Police had passed the matter to their Suffolk colleagues, who approached the situation with notably different energy. One evening, as my mother and I watched television in her bedroom, a gentle tap at the front door announced their arrival.

Peering through the curtained window in the door, I saw a petite female officer in uniform, looking up with what I could only describe as sad spaniel eyes—gentle, almost apologetic. I opened the door.

"I have to let you in because you've such an amicable face," I told her, attempting to defuse the official nature of her visit with humor.

She smiled, explaining she needed to see that my mother was safe and well-cared for. I led her through to the bedroom, where mum greeted her with evident pleasure, responding to the officer's questions with smiles and affirmations.

"Are you alright?" the officer asked Angela directly.

"Yes, yes," mother responded with unexpected clarity.

The officer turned to me. "I can see she's fine. You won't be hearing from us anymore!"

With those simple words, the official pursuit ended. The system retreated from our lives after verifying Angela Webb's basic well-being. The policewoman's report would make its way back to Cambridge authorities, effectively closing the case from a law enforcement perspective. Cambridge Adult Social Services might harbor different opinions, but without police backing, their options for intervention were severely limited.

Freed from the immediate threat of separation, we established our new routines. Angela's physical condition began improving almost immediately. The bedsores that had plagued her at Midfield Lodge started healing once she was no longer confined to a pressure mattress. The wounds on her feet, which I continued to treat using Addenbrooke's specialist's advice about circulation exercises, gradually closed.

Most dramatically, addressing her severe constipation—a problem the care home had either missed or ignored—transformed her comfort and willingness to eat. The woman they had placed on palliative care, declaring she had months to live, was now accepting small meals and showing increasing alertness.

I connected with Suffolk Social Services, approaching them not as adversaries but as potential allies in mum's care. Their response proved refreshingly different from our Cambridge experience. A social worker visited, assessing our needs without judgment about how we had arrived in their jurisdiction. She arranged practical supports—incontinence pads, special bedding, and equipment advice—that made daily care more manageable.

Through her recommendations, I established a relationship with a local care agency. They assigned Lisa, who lived just around the corner, to provide daily support.

As winter turned to spring, our world expanded cautiously. The postman became a welcome daily connection to the outside world. Lisa, our carer, brought practical assistance, conversation, and community news that prevented us from becoming isolated.

The difference between institutional care and home care revealed itself in countless small ways. Angela could eat when hungry rather than when scheduled. She could watch **her** television programs rather than whatever was playing.

"Philip," my mother said one evening as I adjusted her pillows before bedtime, her voice surprisingly clear and present. "Thank you."

Those two words—rare in their coherence and devastating in their simplicity—contained everything. She knew what had happened, what I had done. Despite her cognitive limitations, she recognized the fundamental shift in her circumstances and its meaning. In that moment of connection, the months of planning, the stress of execution, the constant vigilance of our new life—all of it found justification.

We had stood our ground, not through confrontation but through determined withdrawal. We had claimed the right to define care on our own terms. And while I harbored no illusions about the challenges ahead—my mother's condition would inevitably decline, resources would be tested, and my own stamina would face increasing demands—we had secured something precious: the autonomy to face those challenges together, according to values and priorities we determined, not those imposed by distant authorities with clipboards and assessment forms.

As spring blossoms appeared in neighboring gardens, I allowed myself to believe that we had not merely escaped a system but had established an alternative—a reminder that care is not primarily a medical protocol or administrative category but a profound expression of human connection. In our modest house near the Suffolk coast, we were not merely standing our ground; we were reclaiming the fundamental territory of family love against the encroachment of institutional efficiency.

Chapter 9:

Final Days:
July 2019

J uly heat pressed against the windows of our Lowestoft home. Eight months had passed since our great escape —eight months of quiet triumph as Angela flourished under home care. Her bedsores healed, the wounds on her feet closed, and she had regained a modest appetite. The dire predictions of Cambridge S.S. had been proven wrong through the simple application of attentive care.

Yet, as July progressed, subtle shifts in her condition became impossible to ignore. Her periods of wakefulness shortened, and her responses became more delayed. One morning, I entered her room to find her hands moving restlessly across the duvet, her body shifting with discomfort, though she couldn't articulate what troubled her.

"Something's not right," I told Lisa, our carer when she arrived for her morning visit.

She observed Angela for several minutes, her experienced eyes noting the changes in breathing pattern and the unusual restlessness. "I think you should call the doctor," she advised quietly.

The GP arrived that afternoon; his bag weathered from countless similar visits to countless similar bedsides. He gently examined my mother, his stethoscope moving across her chest. At the same time, his eyes cataloged various symptoms

"I think we need to make her more comfortable," he said, the careful euphemism hanging in the air between us.

From his bag, he produced a vial of morphine and administered a small dose—two milligrams to ease her discomfort without overwhelming her system that had never known stronger medication than aspirin. I watched as the lines of tension in her face gradually softened, her breathing becoming less labored.

Before leaving, he wrote a prescription. "You'll need more," he explained, "and I'll arrange for a community nurse to visit regularly to administer it. They'll have a red medical bag with everything necessary."

The next day, I took his prescription to the local pharmacy. The pharmacist, studied it carefully before disappearing into the back. She returned with a box containing morphine vials.

When the doctor returned to check on my mother, he discovered the pharmacy's critical error—they had provided 10mg doses instead of the prescribed 2mg. He gave a sigh calling the blunder "third world" as he struggled to extract the correct dose from the overly concentrated vials.

"This is not right," he muttered, drawing out a tiny portion of the syringe. "It should have been two milligrams so that you can load it straight away." His frustration was palpable as he performed the delicate calibration that should have been unnecessary.

Despite this complication, the system functioned as promised. A community nurse arrived with the distinctive red medical bag. She arranged the vials, syringes, and documentation in the bag, leaving it accessible for subsequent visits.

One evening, noticing another change in her restlessness, I called for the nurse. Instead, paramedics arrived—a staffing decision I hadn't been consulted about. They entered with the peculiar blend of efficiency and compassion that characterizes first responders, moving directly to Angela's bedside to assess her condition.

After their examination, one took me aside in the living room. His voice lowered, and he delivered the news with practiced gentleness: "You need to know your mother's got not long to live. She could go at any moment."

"Yes, I know that," I replied, the knowledge already settled in my bones.

"You need to be prepared," he added, as though I might have misunderstood.

I nodded, recognizing the well-intentioned warning and its inadequacy. How does one "prepare" for such a moment? What preparation could possibly suffice? Nevertheless, I thanked him, and they departed with promises to relay information to the nursing team.

Days passed in the peculiar suspended animation that surrounds imminent loss. I maintained our routines— morning care, afternoon reading, evening television—while watching for each subtle change. Lisa continued her twice-daily visits, providing not just physical care but the emotional sustenance of shared vigilance.

Then came what would be our final evening together. The day had been unremarkable—Angela had sipped a little tea, dozed frequently, and stirred at the sound of familiar television programs. I had been in the kitchen preparing a simple dinner for myself when some instinct drew me to check on her.

Standing in the doorway, I looked toward her bed. Angela's head had fallen slightly to one side on the pillow, her gaze fixed on some distant point beyond the room. Her eyes, usually mobile even in rest, remained utterly still, focused on emptiness with unsettling intensity.

A cold certainty washed through me: she's gone.

I couldn't bring myself to enter the room. The threshold between living and watching over the dead seemed impossible to cross. Instead, I backed away, returning to the kitchen, where I reached for the telephone with trembling hands. I dialed Steve Midgley, senior pastor of Christchurch Cambridge, a spiritual anchor through many storms.

"My mother's gone," I said, when he answered, my voice sounding foreign to my own ears. "I'm on my own."

His response came with immediate compassion. He offered to pray for us both there and then—a thread of connection and comfort across the distance. As his voice provided rhythms of familiar faith, I moved to the drinks cabinet and poured myself a generous measure of brandy, seeking the numbing embrace of alcohol to steady my mind which beckoned to go out of control.

Aware of my own heartbeat continuing its relentless rhythm, aware of the impossible gap that had opened between us, I called Lisa.

Despite the late hour, her response was immediate. "I'm coming," she said, without hesitation.

She arrived within minutes and entered the bedroom with the calm confidence I couldn't muster. She approached Angela's body, gently closing the eyelids that had remained fixed in their final gaze. The simple human gesture transformed the scene—mum now appeared peaceful rather than absent, as though merely sleeping.

Lisa moved with practiced efficiency, making necessary calls to authorities while I sat numbly in the living room, the half-finished brandy warming in my glass. Through her actions, the machinery of death's administration began turning—the official verification, the documentation, the transition from person to paperwork.

Two nurses arrived to register the death, their quiet professionalism a stark contrast to my disordered emotions. They confirmed what was already known, recording the time and circumstances with meticulous care. Throughout this process, Lisa remained by my side, her steady presence a counterweight to my untethered grief.

"We need to arrange the funeral," she said gently when the nurses had gone. "Do you have her policy information?"

I searched frantically through mother's documents, but shock had scrambled my organizational abilities. Despite knowing she had funeral insurance, I couldn't locate the policy details. Lisa, recognizing my distress, took practical action.

"I'll call the Co-op funeral directors," she said. "They can help us sort everything out."

Near midnight, representatives from the funeral home arrived. They moved through our house with quiet respect, their voices hushed, their movements deliberate. I watched as they prepared to take mother's body, transforming our home back into a house, with their careful removal of her physical presence.

As they departed with my mother, that July night pressed against me with overwhelming suffocating intensity.

Eight months exactly since our journey from Cambridge, the circle had closed. I had fulfilled my promise to her and to myself—she had died not in an institution but at home, under my care, with dignity intact.

The emptiness left behind seemed both vast and precise. The bed where she had lain, the chair where I had sat reading to her, the telly she would no longer face, each ordinary object now radiated absence. The house, so carefully prepared for her comfort, now seemed excessive in its accommodation of just one person.

In the following days, the practical matters of death provided the necessary structure. Lisa, sad she wasnt to be buried in Lowestoft, helped arrange the funeral in Cambridge, where my mother would rejoin my father in the plot prepared for them both. My son Austin returned for the ceremony, supported by Joel, who collected him from the station.

The service at the Huntington Road Cemetery united fragments of our scattered lives—church friends from Cambridge, family connections long dormant but awakened by the finality of death. Angela was the final one to die in her generation, the end of an era, her body returned to the city she had known most of her life, though her final months had been spent in exile of my making.

As summer continued its progression toward autumn, I began the slow work of reconstruction. The bedroom that had been hers remained untouched at first, too laden with memory for immediate repurposing. The medical equipment —the hoist, the specialized bed, the supplies—stood as artifacts of a battle both won and lost.

The victory had been in those eight months—in the healing of her bedsores, in the fish and chips by the sea, in the freedom from institutional constraints. The loss was absolute and inevitable, yet somehow softened by the knowledge that it had happened on our terms, not those dictated by distant authorities with forms and protocols.

In quiet moments, I sometimes caught myself listening for sounds from her room—the rustle of bedclothes, the soft rhythm of breathing—before remembering. Grief eased from dramatic waves into these small moments of forgetting followed by remembering, each recollection a new experience of loss.

Yet, alongside grief grew a quiet certainty that we had done the impossible. Against the machinery of social services, against medical pronouncements, against the inertia of institutional care, we had carved out a space where my mother could live her final months with dignity. The system designed to process rather than nurture had been, in our small way, successfully challenged.

On her final night, as her consciousness ebbed, my mother was surrounded not by shift workers and institutional routines but by the familiar scents and sounds of home. The room where she died had been prepared with love rather than professional detachment. The hands that closed her eyes belonged to someone who knew her name and history.

In the end, perhaps that is all any of us can hope for—not immortality, not even a good death in any objective sense, but simply the right to die among those who truly know us, in a place where our preferences matter, our identity remains intact until the final breath.

Angela Webb's last journey had been from Cambridge to Lowestoft, a geographical shift that represented a far more significant transition—from being a case to be managed to being a person to be loved. Her final destination was Cambridge again, but she returned transformed by those intervening months of freedom, carrying with her the victory we had won together.

As July gave way to August, I stood at her graveside, placing flowers beside the freshly turned earth. The headstone would eventually bear both their names—Angela and her husband Sam, reunited in this plot of Cambridge soil after their separate journeys through illness and care.

"We did it, Mum," I whispered to the quiet earth. "We brought you home."

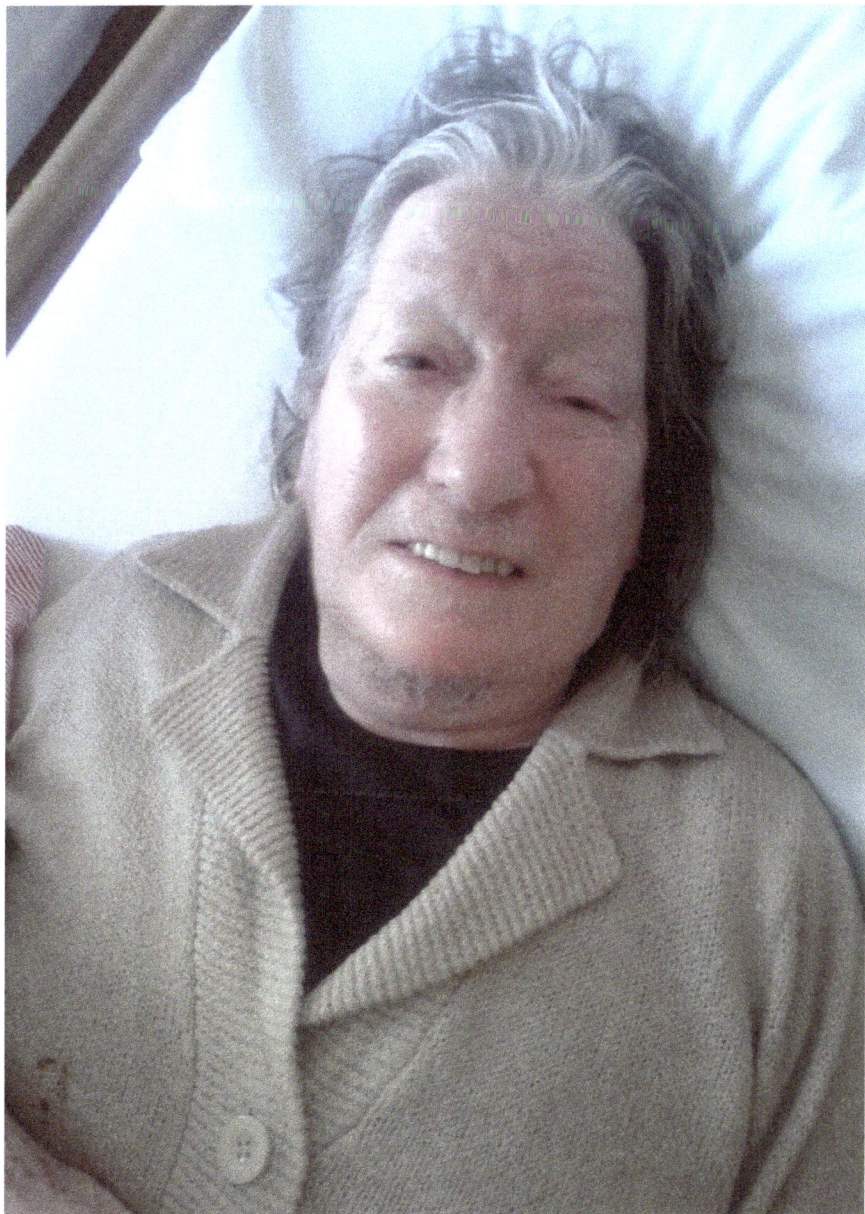

Anglela looking up seeing her son was there. You'll be meeting Jesus I said and you'll be coming with me, she replied!

Chapter 10:

Coming Home To Cambridge

The morning sun hung low in the sky, its pale light filtering through the trees as we began our final journey together, I chose to sit beside my mum's coffin as it began its 86 mile journey along the A143, from the most easterly town in the UK, to the spires and steeples of Cambridge, its river punts moored up along the quiet banks of the Cam, the town of my birth, the ancient stone walls a testament to the enduring power of faith and tradition.

But on this day, as the funeral procession wound its way through the long entrance to the Cremation and Burial Cemetery, the weight of a different kind of history pressed down upon us - the history of a life lived in service to others, and a love that had endured through the darkest of times.

At the head of the procession, the hearse carried Angela's body - the earthly vessel that had once housed her indomitable spirit, now still and silent in the face of eternity. Behind it, a small group of mourners followed on foot - friends and family members who had gathered to pay their final respects, and to shoulder me as I bid farewell to a woman who had touched so many lives.

As we arrived at the gates of the Cemetery I felt a sense of coming home - a deep, abiding connection to the place that had shaped my mother's life, and my own. It was here, among the ancient headstones and gnarled oak trees, that she would find her final resting place - beside the husband who had been her rock and her refuge, through all the trials and triumphs of their long and happy marriage.

The grave had been prepared in advance, a simple plot marked out with a temporary wooden cross. But as I stood there, watching as the casket was lowered into the ground, I couldn't help but feel a sense of finality - a recognition that this was the end of a journey that had begun so many years ago, in a tiny cottage near the edge of the river cam surrounded by great pillars of learning, spires and steeples, bells a ringing across the city and the sound of owls hooting in the night.

"Ashes to ashes, dust to dust." The words of the priest hung in the air, a solemn reminder of the impermanence of all things. But even as the tears began to fall, I could feel a sense of peace settling over me - a quiet, centered stillness that seemed to emanate from somewhere deep within, a strength that lies hidden, sometimes dormant but nonetheless saves me from falling.

For I knew that my mother's legacy would live on - not in the cold, hard ground of the cemetery, but in the hearts and minds of all those who had known and loved her. It was a legacy of kindness and compassion, of strength and resilience in the face of adversity. And it was a legacy that I would carry with me, now and always, as I made my way through the world without her.

As the service drew to a close, I felt a hand on my shoulder - a gentle, reassuring touch that seemed to anchor me in the present moment. I turned to see Joel, his face etched with sympathy, but also that familiar glint in his eye saying you're gonna be alright brov, we're here.

"I Recognised your son immediately at the train station," he said, his voice soft but deliberate. "Everyone will meet for the gathering at the hotel, don't worry, Richard (Newman) has arranged it all. I have to get back to Sarah," Joel's wife was expecting their third child, she gave birth 6 days later to Ezra, a wonderful baby boy.

I nodded, my throat tight with emotion. In the midst of my grief, I had completely forgotten about aranging a wake, somewhere for those closest to me to come together, to share their memories and to offer their support.

As we made our way to the hotel, I couldn't help but marvel at the outpouring of love and compassion that surrounded me. From church friends who had dropped everything to be by my side, to the staff at the hotel who had it not been for my sweet and long standing friend Richard, would not have gone above and beyond to make us feel welcome at such short notice, it was a testament to the impact my mother had on me that showed how I made such great friends.

Outside overlooking the hotel golf course a private table had been set aside for our group - a quiet, intimate space where we could gather and chat freely to one another and unwind from what is always a solemn, emotionally charged occasion. As I stepped through onto the terrace I was struck by the sight of familiar faces, people who were and still are a part of my life. Their faces bore the mark of compassion and empathy, one that comes to us all, yet I still could not take in what was happening, I could not believe I was at my mothers own funeral- it all seemed so unreal. It was as if I was being led through some interdimensional dream and my mum was still alive somewhere, she who brought me into this world, who clothed and fed me and showed me love, who helped to support me through the darkest of times...but its not a dream its all very real, and the world from now on is going to be a very, very different place.

At the center of the large open roof terrace a long table had been laid out with refreshments - sandwiches and cakes, tea and coffee, all arranged with the kind of care and attention to detail that spoke volumes about the sort of people and the occasion that had brought us all together.

As I made my way around, shaking hands and exchanging hugs with those who had come to support me I couldn't help but feel a sense of gratitude - a deep, abiding thankfulness for the incredible network of support that had sustained me through the most difficult period of my life.

But it was a comment from that man again, Richard Newman that truly captured the essence of the day - a wry observation that seemed to encapsulate the unique nature of our story, and the bond that had brought us all together.

"You know," he said, a hint of a smile playing around the corners of his mouth, "I've never been to a funeral where the son took his own mother hostage."

For a moment, there was a stunned silence - a breath of disbelief that hung heavy in the air. But then, as if on cue, the air erupted in laughter - a cathartic release of emotion that seemed to break the tension and bring us all closer together.

It was a moment that I would never forget - a reminder that even in the midst of the deepest sorrow, there was still room for joy and laughter and the kind of irreverent humor that had always been such an important part of my relationship with my mother.

As the day wore on, and the guests began to file away, I found myself alone - trying to reflect on this incredible journey that brought us here.

It had been five long years since my mother's passing - five years of grief and healing, of coming to terms with the loss that had shattered my world and left me adrift in a sea of uncertainty. But it had also been five years of growth and discovery, of learning to navigate the complexities of the care system and to fight for what I believed in, no matter the cost.

Looking back now, I realized that I had needed that time - a period of reflection and introspection, in which to process the incredible events that had shaped my life and my mother's final days. It had taken me this long to feel ready to share our story - to put into words the love and devotion that had sustained us through the most difficult of times, and the incredible resilience that had allowed us to triumph in the face of overwhelming odds.

But as I sat, surrounded by the memories of the past and the promise of the future, I knew that the time had finally come - that I was ready to speak out, to share our story with the world and to shine a light on the flaws and the failings of a system that had let us down when we needed it most.

For though the care system had been designed to protect and support those in need, I had seen firsthand how often it fell short - how the cold, clinical calculations of bureaucracy could never truly capture the depth of human emotion and the power of familial love.

In the end, my mother's story was a testament to the unbreakable bond between a mother and son - a reminder that no matter the obstacles that lay ahead, no matter the trials and tribulations that we might face, the love and devotion of a family could never be truly extinguished.

As I looked out the window at the setting sun, its warm, golden rays casting a soft glow over the city that had been my home for so long, I felt a sense of peace settling over me - a deep, abiding sense of closure and acceptance, of knowing that I had done everything in my power to honor my mother's memory and to carry on her legacy of love and compassion.

And though there would always be a part of me that wondered what might have been - that questioned whether things could have turned out differently, if only the system had been more responsive to our needs - I knew that dwelling on the past would do nothing to change the reality of our situation.

Instead, I resolved to look to the future - to use the lessons that I had learned and the strength that I had gained to make a difference in the lives of others, to fight for a world in which no one would ever have to endure the kind of pain and heartache that my mother and I had faced.

For in the end, that was the true legacy of Angela Webb - not the disease that had ravaged her body, nor the indignities that she had suffered in her final days, but the love and compassion that she had inspired in all those who knew her, and the unwavering ~determination to make the world a better place, one small act of kindness at a time.

As I recall the faces around that table - the faces of the people who knew of the torment at the beginning, the heartbreaks and pressures that cut into one's soul, but yet had stood by us through the darkest of times, I knew that no matter what the future might hold, no matter where the road might take me, I would always carry a piece of them with me - a reminder of the incredible power of human connection, and the unbreakable bonds of love and family that had brought us to this place.

With a deep breath and a silent prayer to our Lord and maker, I stepped out into the world - ready to face whatever challenges lay ahead, armed with the strength and resilience that comes now from knowing I'm not afraid in this new strange, divided world, believing that one day in some other place my mother and I shall meet again in the knowledge that God's love, that which shone so strong through her would always be a part of my guiding light, now and forever until the end of my days.

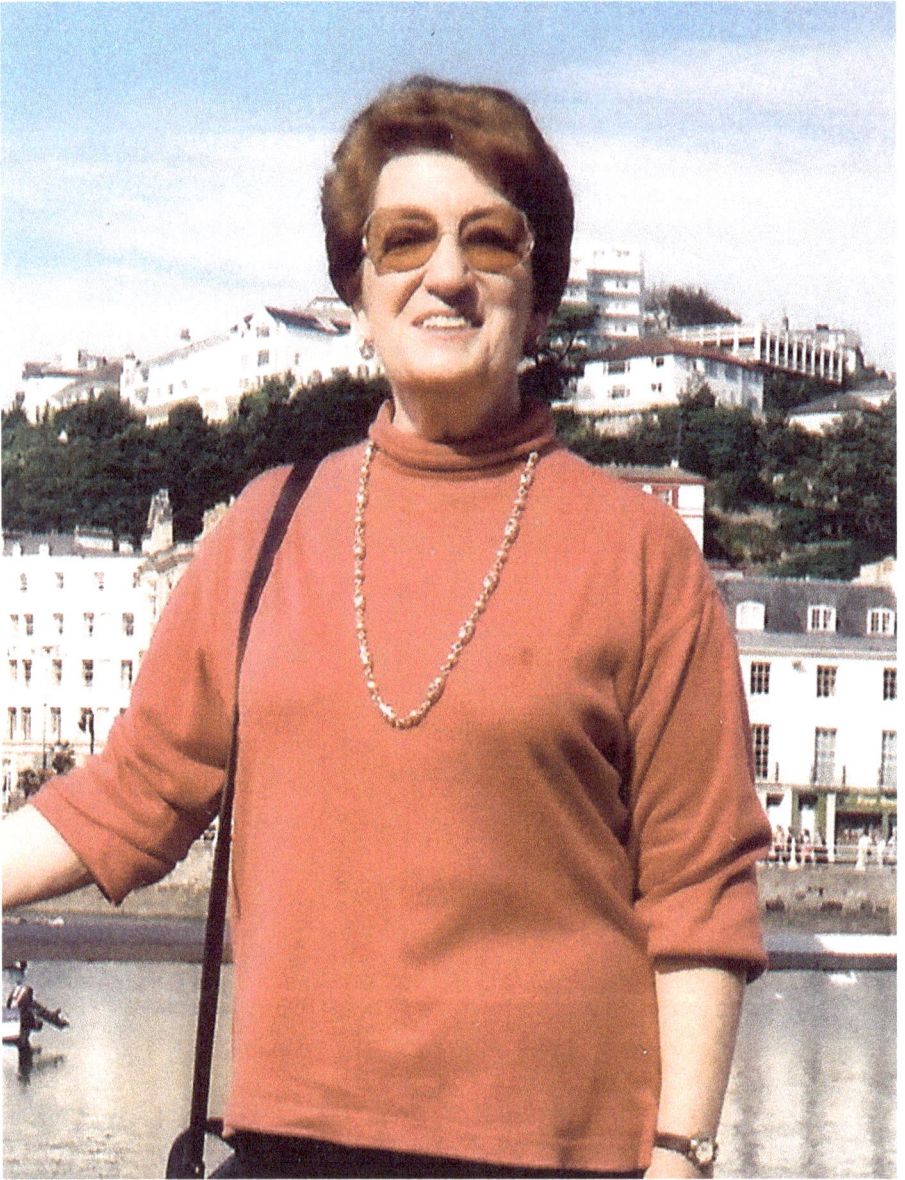

Angela Webb, 2nd March 1933 ~~~ 31st July 2019. Death has no hold over love.

110

www.ingramcontent.com/pod-product-compliance
Lightning Source LLC
Chambersburg PA
CBHW050843270326
41930CB00019B/3446